What People Say About Abby

~ Susan, Houston, Texas

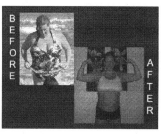

"For many years, I did not have good knowledge of food and nutrition though I thought I knew what healthy eating was. It wasn't until I had gotten serious about lifting weights that I made a plea for muscle definition. That's when I became acquainted with Abby who was very kind to share her knowledge of nutrition and give me suggestions on how to change my diet for results. After taking her suggestions, I had a significant weight loss over the summer! That's when I realized how important it is to be conscious of what and when I eat it. I am so grateful for Abby. She is very passionate about helping people get in shape and achieve their fitness goals." **~60 total pounds lost**

~ Jess, Albuquerque, New Mexico

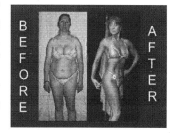

"I received much support with Abby. She helped me with my food intake when I was overweight, and basically on a starvation diet, a couple of years back that gave me terrible headaches and dizzy spells. She has also supported me through all my goals from weight loss in 2008 to my stage competition in July 2010 when I competed for figure athlete. She has been a great friend!" **~60 total pounds lost.**

~ Cassandra, Sierra Vista, Arizona

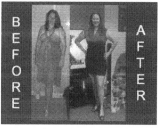

"I am a working mother of two and as if that isn't enough, I am trying to train for a triathlon to help me lose weight. I was having a hard time finding energy for my workouts. I was so hungry, but ended up overeating and not seeing any results. Abby helped me by giving me great advice on my diet and ideas for meals to help me maintain the proper balance I needed while trying to train and lose weight. I learned how to balance starchy carbs and essential fats. She worked very closely with me until I got the hang on how to plan and balance my meals. I have learned that 'fat' is not the enemy and very necessary to weight loss!! I recommend Abby because she is knowledgeable, supportive, and very complete!" **~60 total pounds lost.**

~ Amber, Littleton, Colorado

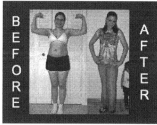

"I had always been fit before having my little ones 13 months apart. Getting back in shape was hard for me and I had to be really motivated and dedicated to not use the kids or other things as an excuse to miss workouts. Abby has been a real help in motivating me and helping me stay on track. She is always so friendly and encouraging and always has great ideas and suggestions I can use in my daily diet and exercise routine. It's great having someone who leads by example and is there to keep me staying accountable." **~25 total pounds lost.**

~ Dawn-Marie, Henderson, Nevada

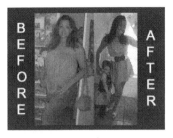

"I am a mother of 3 girls and have decided to focus on myself and have been dedicated on workouts and eating right. I came across Abby in a fitness group. I was having trouble losing weight and was stuck. Abby gave me GREAT help on my meals which I applied religiously and have stuck with it. It was hard at first, but she's such a great inspiration and great motivator. Great reason I recommend Abby! I've learned so much by her training and her meals, and I learn new things every day from her." ~50 total pounds lost.

~ Candice, Eglin Air Force Base, Florida

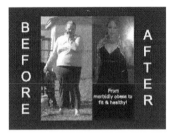

"After seeing three different doctors and two different nutritionists over a two year span, I still had no idea what foods I needed to be eating to lose weight and eat clean and healthy. The two doctors would simply tell me to eat under 1,200 calories a day. One even told me to eat a low carb diet. The nutritionist would leave me with, 'Don't eat any sweets and most of your diet should be vegetables.' None of that told me how to really eat healthy and how to feed my family healthy meals. Then Abby gave me advice that actually made sense. She made it easy to understand. She was able to tell me what foods were the best ones to eat to reach my goals, and best of all she gave me advice that I could apply to feeding my family. Within a week of using her guidelines I was starting to feel healthier and it was wonderful. Abby has also given many exercises that I can do within my physical capabilities that have really helped me get stronger and leaner. Abby really takes the time to care about the people she helps." ~120 total pounds lost.

~ Melinda, Bronx, New York

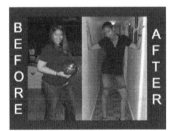

"A few years ago, I finally decided to take back my health and started on a journey to losing weight. About two months later, I discovered an internet group that was geared for those serious into getting fit and healthy. This was exactly what I was looking for. In that group I met Abby, a wonderful knowledgeable woman of all things fitness. She directed me on a right path of health and nutrition that I would not have gotten to on my own. She helped give me a better knowledge of foods that would benefit my body and recommended exercises that were specific to my needs. I have known her for several months now and can honestly say I value her advice, encouragement, and support that continues to give because I know she offers it with passion and love she has for every woman to be their very best." ~70 total pounds lost.

~ Janet, Portland, Oregon

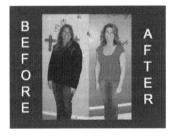

"Losing weight was one of the most difficult things I ever tried, but it got so much easier once I dug deep within myself. My will plus Abby's help brought success. Quick fixes never last, but habits do! That is exactly what Abby taught me – good nutrition habits. Now that I have built them, I sometimes look back and wonder how it was ever so difficult." ~75 total pounds lost

Please see www.AbbyCampbellOnline.com for more testimonies.

One Size Does NOT Fit All Diet Plan

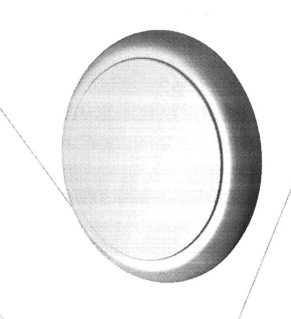

One Size Does NOT Fit All Diet Plan

Meal Planning That Will Boost Your
Metabolism, Break Through
Plateaus, and Help You Achieve
Maximum Fat Loss Today!

Body Works *Publications*

Author Abby Campbell, BSc, SFN, SSN, CPT

Editor Ann Phillips
Consultant Editor Nick Castrellon
Cover Illustrator Derek Murphy
Foreword by Isaac Warbrick, Ph.D.

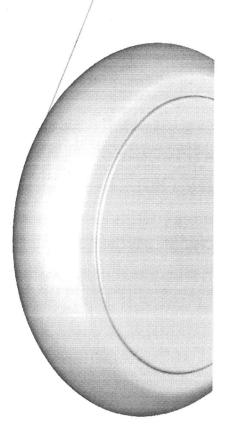

One Size Does NOT Fit All Diet Plan: Meal Planning That Will Boost Your Metabolism, Break Through Plateaus, and Help You Achieve Maximum Fat Loss Today!

ISBN-13: 978-1-939015-00-6
1. Health   2. Nutrition   3. Weight Loss   4. Diet

Library of Congress Control Number: 2012945998

Version 1:1
First Printing, January 2013 (paperback edition, 7" x 10")

Publisher:

Body Works
Publications

Body Works Publications
301 W. Main Ave. #44, Gastonia, NC 28053

Author: Abby Campbell
Editor: Ann Phillips
Consultant Editor: Nick Castrellon
Cover Illustrator Derek Murphy
Foreword by Isaac Warbrick, Ph.D.

For more information, including quantity discounts, about *One Size Does NOT Fit All Diet Plan*, please visit AbbyCampbellOnline.com.

Acknowledgments

I can honestly say this book is long overdue, but I know that all good things come to those who wait. It is just the beginning of many good things to come, yet I would like to express my gratitude to all those who have helped shape me and the knowledge shared within the pages here in this book.

First and foremost, I want to thank my family, especially my beloved husband and girls. Rob, you have had to put up with a lot during my training, research, and writing. You have been my biggest fan even when I spent many countless nights behind closed doors in my office while leaving you to be alone. Carter and Mattie, thank you for being super supportive. Mattie, you have even given me a run for my money in the gym while showing me up has been your specialty and a great challenge for me.

Thank you to my "other" girls – all the wonderful ladies who continue to trust me with advice, menu plans, and training. You have been extremely supportive. Your awesome transformation in body, mind, and overall health are extraordinaire, yet you have helped me as a believer in all things great. A special thank you goes out to my greatest supporters – Cassandra, Tricia, Jessica, and Dawn-Marie. Oh! I can't forget to thank my "guy" friends too – Nick, Jimmie, and Doug.

I also want to thank those who have taught me great nutrition and fitness principles to stick by: Dr. John Berardi, Alwyn Cosgrove, Jeff Kuh, Darin Steen, Tom Venuto, Dr. Isaac Warbrick, and Chad Waterbury.

To my dear friends, Ann Phillips and Nick Castrellon, I thank you for taking the time to review and edit *One Size Does NOT Fit All Diet Plan* before it went to press. It takes a careful eye and great intelligence to incorporate change for the better.

This book has been a rewarding journey for me to write as I hope it will be a rewarding journey for those who will read it and put the great principles within it to use. My only goal is to help those in need. Education is the key to all things life changing.

This book is dedicated to all those who face the challenge of living a healthy lifestyle. You are my heroes as you continue to battle the storm of bad information from media, advertisements, and even those you trust such as doctors and dieticians. Continue to ride out the downpour because you will find the peace and calm. Once you're there, no whirlwind or gust will overtake you again.

THRIVE TO THE END!

About the Author

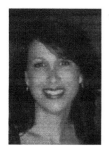

Abby Campbell is a professional fitness and sports nutritionist, personal trainer, and author of the *One Size Does NOT Fit All Diet Plan* series.

As the proprietor of 911 Body ResQ in the Charlotte region of North Carolina, a fitness and nutrition consulting company, Abby has worked primarily with overweight and obese women. In 2009, she launched www.911BodyResQ.com where she took her business online due to many requests from women in weight loss and fitness forums that she administrated and moderated. Through her popularity, she is known as one of America's favorite weight loss experts. She has also been a director's consultant for the YMCA since 2006.

Since a small girl, Abby knew she wanted to be a writer. Her teachers always titled her as "Most Creative" with short stories, and her political English professor encouraged her to co-publish books on research she had done for college papers. It wasn't until she got involved with weight loss and fitness forums that she found her passion for writing for the public. Due to Abby's concern for the growing weight crisis in America, she wanted to reach more people with nutrition truth. She began blogging and writing articles for online fitness sites and e-zines. Her email would then get filled with questions that took up much of her day, so she wrote and distributed free e-books to satisfy those wanting more knowledge about nutrition and healthy living. Current statistics indicate that 80 percent of the 75 million dieters in the United States want an inexpensive, low-cost, and home-based plan for losing weight. Due to these statistics, Abby finally decided to publish her nutrition plans to fulfill the need of the masses. Her book is the only book on the market that provides a personalized approach.

Abby has a Bachelor of Science degree in business administration, professional certifications in both fitness and sports nutrition with International Sports Sciences Association, as well as certification in personal training with Athletic Certification Training Commission.

In her spare time, Abby likes to hike, garden, and read. She resides in the Charlotte, North Carolina, area and has been married for 20 years with three grown daughters, one of which is autistic. Abby is also a 19 year cancer survivor.

How to Contact the Author

The company founded by Abby Campbell provides full consulting services on a first come, first serve basis. Helpful articles may also be found on her website. Requests for further information, as well as inquiries about the author's availability for group consulting services and book signings, should be directed to her at the address below. Readers of this book are also encouraged to contact the author with comments and ideas for future editions.

Body Works Publications
301 W. Main Ave. #44
Gastonia, NC 28053
Tel: 704-215-4376

Abby Campbell
911 Body ResQ

Email: Abby@911BodyResQ.com

Websites: AbbyCampbellOnline.com & 911BodyResQ.com

Book information: AbbyCampbellOnline.com

Facebook Fan Pages:
www.facebook.com/Abby.911BodyResQ
www.facebook.com/FANPAGE.911BodyResQ

Facebook Support Group:
www.facebook.com/groups/BurnFatLoseWeight/

Facebook Support Group for Book Buyers Only (NEW):
www.facebook.com/groups/AbbyCampbellDietPlanning/

LinkedIn: www.linkedin.com/in/abbycampbell
Pinterest: www.pinterest.com/911abbycampbell/
Twitter: www.twitter.com/911BodyResQ
Yelp: www.abbycampbell.yelp.com

Supporting the Hungry

Proper nutrition is important for all people. Receiving appropriate vitamins, minerals, and phytonutrients through a proper and balanced diet are extremely important for optimal health. The book you hold in your hands is a source to help you on your journey to good health. Unfortunately, not everyone has the means to educate themselves. In fact, many don't even have the means to feed themselves and must rely on others for help. Therefore, I have pledged a portion of the proceeds for each book sold to the homeless in my local area – Charlotte, North Carolina.

Since 1938, Charlotte Rescue Mission (CRM) has served the poor and homeless. They are an organization that intensified its focus on homelessness by addressing the connection between homelessness and substance abuse. They provide nourishing meals, safe shelters, and long-term (100-130 days) recovery programs to the hungry, homeless, and hurting. They not only help those that bring no luggage, but help each participant on their "baggage." Each person that walks through CRM's doors receives help to be transformed from the "inside-out." Forty-five percent of their men and 74 percent of their women complete their programs when the national average is 18 percent. One year later, 75 percent of their program graduates are still sober compared to the national average of 25 percent.

Money is frequently tight with many non-profit organizations, especially during an economy that is hurting. Food and nutrition can often be shortchanged. This is why I want to donate a portion of the proceeds from *One Size Does NOT Fit All Diet Plan* to CRM. I want to ensure that they are able to help these hurting souls find the recovery they need which begins with feeding their bellies. Thank you for helping me support the hungry, homeless, and hurting.

For more information on CRM's excellent programs, please visit www.CharlotteRescueMission.org .

Abby Campbell

Foreword

> ## "Habits first, results second."

It's ironic that in our modern world, the only thing matching the ever-accelerating pace of work and life is the ever decreasing pace of the average human metabolism. Come to think of it, the only aspect of our physical selves which seems to be advancing in parallel to modern living is our waistlines. Thing is, the cure to these ills is well-known. You don't need an advanced degree in medicine, nutrition, or physiology to know that eating well and a little exercise will solve most of the health issues plaguing you, me, him, and that girl over there *(hopefully you're not reading this in an empty room)*.

Sadly, obtaining correct information about weight loss these days is often a matter of un-learning nutritional here-say, than actually learning anything new, ground-breaking, or Twitter-worthy. Food marketers are notoriously good at appealing to the consumer *(that's you by the way)* by offering an endless variety of options – the 'you're bound to find something you like' approach. One of the biggest solutions to this barrage of food choices however is almost always prescribed en mass: the one-size-fits-all approach to health and weight loss. I know it's hard to tell by reading this, but I'm a 6'5" 220 pound male and common sense dictates that a small leafy salad with a hobbit-sized piece of salmon is not going to feed my inner-Chrysler!

Abby Campbell takes a much different approach to weight loss and eating well in *One Size Does NOT Fit All Diet Plan*, targeting eating plans directly to the most important person in this world... YOU. From the first few pages, Abby cuts through the fat *(excuse the pun)* so that you know exactly where she's going with this and can already begin to make changes from the first chapter. Rather than basing her program on a particular 'super' food or the teachings of some extreme dietary guru, Abby's program is based on simple and solid dietary principles which make sense – principles that work. Who wants to eat lemons all day anyway?

Abby backs each step of *One Size Does NOT Fit All Diet Plan* with scientific evidence, which really brings peace of mind to those who have struggled through hundreds of fad diets in the past, while also making academic egg heads like me happy.

Lastly, the diagrams, flow charts, and tables that are included make it easy to follow Abby's natural progression from developing a few healthy eating habits, to obtaining the body you want *(and deserve)* with tasty and nutritious food. With a quick glance at the *One Size Does NOT Fit All Diet Plan* blueprint, you'll have countless meal options and ideas at the flick of a page, which you can mix and match to meet your taste, preference, and lifestyle.

It's great to finally see a dietary program that is tailored to the individual. Fittingly, the testimonials within these pages represent a handful of individuals whom Abby has helped to look good, feel great, lose weight, and keep it off. I commend Abby for the many successes she has already had, much of which stem from her ability to personalize the journey toward weight loss and healthy living to each individual, and I am excited to see many more testimonials as a result of her *One Size Does NOT Fit All Diet Plan.*

Isaac Warbrick, Ph.D.
www.wellfactor.net

Dr. Isaac Warbrick is a researcher at Massey University in New Zealand, specializing in exercise physiology and chronic illness. He is also involved in the development of tertiary educational programs to enhance the lifestyles of indigenous people through exercise and nutrition. The husband, and father of two (soon to be three), manages his own health promotion company. He also runs www.wellfactor.net, a website aimed at bringing health and wellness to the masses.

Table of Contents

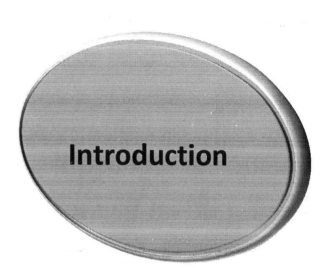

Introduction

An "Individualized" Diet Plan That Works!

My goal for you!

In a world full of confusion due to various diets, magic pills, and misinformation – my goal is to give you dieting techniques and tips based on scientific research and tested on tens of thousands of people. It is even used by holistic professionals, athletes, and figure models throughout the world. My goal is to provide you with a diet, or meal planning system, that is one of the soundest approaches to be applied toward your health and performance endeavors. I also want to show you how you can transform your body into the fit and sexy one you've been longing for. No longer is this diet just for those who have paid big bucks to elite nutrition consultants! When you are feeling healthy and fit, you want to conquer the world. Having you live life to its fullest is my ultimate goal for you. I can and plan to do that by providing you with the best nutrition knowledge available, without the gimmicks. After all, food was never meant to be used as an emotional crutch or lover of the soul. It is meant to fortify your body to live life to its fullest with joy, happiness, and love for others.

> *"Food can be used as a poison or a prescription. Why not use it as a prescription for good health?"*

Introduction

"Beauty is in everything." This quote was made by a famous philosopher named Confucius of the early sixth century, and many try to live their lives on this very quote. In all reality though, it has failed many. It doesn't matter if you're the most compassionate and loving person on the earth. Others still see you for what you are on the exterior. It really isn't fair! Because of that, you have a difficult time when you see yourself in the mirror and the feelings that arise from that are even more intense. Am I right? You know that the way you look on the outside does hold partial responsibility for your happiness, and you may have tried a weight loss diet here or there. It might have been a low-calorie, low-carb, low-fat, or even a starvation diet. You may have even exercised to the point where you thought your heart would drop out. Temptations to "empty out" or pop a few fat burners when no one is looking has probably even crossed your mind. You may even be a cycle dieter moving from dieting and exercising to cravings and binges, only to start over again. No matter what avenue you have taken to lose weight, it may seem that the road is leading you to Nowhere Land. It doesn't have to be so! You can change your health and your body. You can even find energy as well as the sexy body that you're currently covering up.

With the modern age of technology, you have the opportunity to learn about anything you want. Just surf the internet and you'll find tons of information about dieting and exercise. But, have you ever found yourself on information overload? One site will talk about calories and how much you should have if you want to lose weight. Another will talk about how calories don't really matter but the food you eat does. Then there's discussion about macronutrients. Is a high protein diet good for you? Is low-carb the way to go? What about low-fat? South Beach? Atkins? Paleo? On top of that, you're probably asking yourself what supplements you should take and how much exercise you should do. Like a computer running out of memory, your brain starts to short circuit as well.

I completely understand where you're coming from as I was in that place for many years. I not only struggled with weight loss issues, but I also battled with health issues. My health issues lasted for several years while robbing me of my youthful 20s. I want to share with you my story because I am going to follow up with the miracles that took place in my early 30s. These same miracles can be yours too!

My Story

To make a long story short, I was diagnosed with cancer when I was 25 and five months pregnant with my second child. Doctors pleaded with me to abort. Though late-term abortion was against the law at the time, exceptions were made for those with medical necessity. I was one of those cases as my pregnancy and my health were considered "high risk" due to having a progressive form of cancer. Doctors wanted me to terminate my pregnancy so that they could begin treatment before the cancer would invade my body. I was only given five years to live if I didn't terminate. Being the stubborn person I am, and having a great love for my unborn child, I left my fate in the hands of God. I held off on cancer treatment for five months so that I could give birth to my beautiful baby girl. Thankfully, the cancer did not spread, and I had surgery to remove the cancer twice within six months postpartum.

After cancer treatment, I didn't feel well physically for a long time. This also caused depression to set in as I had severe physical pain all the time. Having muscular and nerve pains, as well as optic neuritis, did not make for a fun lifestyle. Being in my 20s, I wanted to have fun and enjoy my children without feeling like the typical older woman. After several years of seeing doctors and having a multitude of tests, I was diagnosed with Multiple Sclerosis (MS). MS is an autoimmune disease that affects the brain and central nervous system due to damage of the myelin sheath which is the protective covering that surrounds nerve cells. Needless to say, I was devastated. How can a young person (me) be struck with two awful diseases in just 3 years? How could life be so unfair?

In the back of my mind, I knew that foods provide nutrients to the body. I began looking at my diet as I was desperate for a cure. In my opinion, my diet seemed to be pretty good. I didn't have too many pre-packaged foods full of preservatives, but I gave those up too. I even gave up some natural starchy carbs like potatoes. I also went "sugar-free." To my surprise, my symptoms were only exacerbated. I felt I was doomed for life! Confusion set in. How could I feel worse when I was doing everything right? It just didn't make any sense.

After three long years of suffering, I finally learned that my sugar-free foods like jams, drink mixes, and gums were actually my enemies as they were artificially sweetened with a man-made chemical called "aspartame." After removing the little bits of processed foods from my diet, especially the ones containing this horrible poison, I felt like a new woman! My pain was gone, and my MS diagnosis was overturned.

Hallelujah for being pain free! Yet, I still struggled as I now had all this extra body fat that came with not being active. Due to stress those several years, my cortisol levels were high which was making me store body fat, particularly belly fat. Because I had never been "fat" before cancer, I was disgusted with myself whenever I passed the mirror. I then did what most American women do and that being diet, diet, and diet more. After losing the weight, I became the master manipulator of my body whenever I needed to lose a little weight. I soon realized that too came with a high price as my thyroid was destroyed in the process of my yo-yo dieting (fat burners, low-carb diets, as well as starvation diets). I would have to work even harder to keep the body fat off.

I can't change what I went through in my 20s, but I believe we all go through certain experiences for one reason or another. We can look at them as negative and hold bitterness throughout life, but I like to find the good that can come from all my obstacles. It was only through my cancer and MS experiences that I found a love for research and sharing. Over the last 15 years, I have done tons of research and now I get to share what I know will help you through your weight and health struggles.

Why this Book?

The reason why I am writing this book is because I want to help you. There are many "diet" books on the market. I've read just about every one of them. I've even used some of those crazy diets myself when I was struggling with body fat. I do believe that the principles in some of those diet books are good. However, there is one flaw in *all* of them. That flaw has to do with the menu plans given. Sure, some have great food sources listed. The problem is that they give the same menus to every single person, and those menus are very vague.

If you think logically, why would a 300 pound man be on the same diet as a 150 pound woman? Sure, they both will lose weight initially living on 1,000 calories or less per day (which is what many diets prescribe). It is usually short-lived for a variety of reasons though. Most likely, someone who is on one of these extremely low calorie diets will fizzle out. They will fizzle out in more ways than one. First, their bodies will get so fatigued that they end up giving up on the diet and binge thereafter because their bodies are screaming for the nutrients it needs. Second, their bodies' immune systems are compromised. These types of diets are what I call "starvation" diets. Have you ever dieted and hit a brick wall where you couldn't lose anymore? You probably wanted to beat your head against the wall because you're doing everything the diet book says to do, yet you stopped losing weight. These "one-size-fits-all" diets are causing your thyroid to slow down. In turn, your weight loss has hit a plateau. The only way you will be able to lose more is by either cutting your calories or exercising more. But, how much more can you do this? These diets create a vicious cycle that wreaks havoc on your body while creating a decline in your metabolism that you may never be able to fix.

I want to share with you some wonderful steps and plans in my book *One Size Does NOT Fit All Diet Plan: Meal Planning That Will Boost Your Metabolism, Break Through Plateaus, and Help You Achieve Maximum Fat Loss*. I will show you how to eat to lose body fat without compromising your metabolism. You will also learn how certain foods along with nutrient timing will help you bust through body fat. In turn, you gain a healthy lifestyle while being able to perform your daily activities throughout life.

How I Got This Information

Like I've mentioned earlier, I've spent years on research. Much of my research has been on exercise and nutrition. I'm no doctor, but I do have some education behind me. I have my bachelors of science degree, but the best education I received was through a variety of other sources. I received several professional certifications. Most importantly is Fitness Nutrition, as well as Sports Nutrition, certifications from International Sports Sciences Association, the leading authority in fitness education. My instructor at the time, and current mentor, is world renowned sports and nutrition expert, Dr. John Berardi of Precision Nutrition. I have also studied many works of other notable fitness and nutrition experts: Alwyn Cosgrove, Jeff Kuh, Darin Steen, Tom Venuto, Dr. Isaac Warbrick, and Chad Waterbury. I have also been coached by some of the best trainers in the world, including Krista Schaus who is also with Precision Nutrition. I have and continue to do research with university and medical journals in the areas of fitness and nutrition, and I am currently being educated to receive my Masters in Natural Health Sciences. In addition, I have been an administrator or moderator for several fitness, nutrition, and weight loss forums over the years. Therefore, I have learned the best from people like you and me. I have seen the struggles of real people, and I've seen and experimented to find what really works.

What's to Come

"Diet" is included in the title of this book. You are not to get the wrong impression here. Dictionary.com defines diet as "the kinds of food that a person, animal, or community habitually eats." If we are *habitually* eating certain kinds of foods, then wouldn't that be long-term or throughout life? A diet is not short-term as other diet books on the market have made it to be. With that being said, you will be learning about a real diet – a lifestyle diet that will keep you healthy as well as rev up your metabolism (not cause it to go into decline as most other diets have you do). With a roaring metabolism, you will be able to lose the unwanted body fat and inches. With a higher metabolism, you will even be able to eat more. Best of all, you'll feel great after learning and incorporating the basic principles of nutrition. Are you ready for physical and mental energy?

You won't find a lot of "fluff" in this book. I know when I was searching for answers, I got very frustrated with all the diet books on the market because they were either full of science that I didn't understand at the time, or they told a gazillion testimonial stories of other folks who succeeded on those diets and without enough information to say how success came about. I just wanted the "meat" so that I could get started quickly. Therefore, I've broken this book down into four parts so that you can get started quickly. For those who want more of the science stuff, I've referenced those parts. You will see superscripted numbers that point to the reference and website (if any) in the Endnotes. For testimonials, you can view videos, see pictures, and read stories on my websites.

The first part of this book is fairly short. It provides information on overweight and obesity statistics. I feel it's important for you to know the seriousness of this epidemic as it will hopefully urge you to use the nutrition principles I've outlined in this book. There is also a chapter that goes further in depth on why "one-size-fits-all" diet plans do not work. It includes the reasons why many licensed dieticians are not educated though many have their masters of science degrees. If you want to quickly get to the meat of the book, then skip this part for now. Just move onto the second part, and come back and read it later.

The heart of the book comes with Part II. You will find your meat here and will definitely get filled. The pillars of good nutrition are discussed here, but this part is also broken down into smaller parts depending on your nutritional age. Depending on what you know about these pillars, as well as what you do with them and how consistent you are, will determine your nutritional age and what you will use in this section. Here is where you will figure your intentions and set your course of action.

How to set you up for success is discussed in Part III with kitchen details. How to stock your kitchen with the right foods and gear is discussed, but the most important topic will be how to prepare for success. Preparation is the key to success with just about anything in life, and it is extremely important when it comes to weight loss and living a healthy lifestyle. Steps will be given for your preparation. Moreover, would a diet book be complete without some recipes? This part also offers some wonderful healthy yet simple recipes for snacks, breakfasts, lunches, and dinners.

Part IV gets into nutritional supplements. Necessary supplements are discussed as well as supplements for special needs.

Finally, you will find a tremendous amount of helpful resources in the back of the book. Not only does it include an appendix, glossary, index, and endnotes full of references. It also includes some recommended reading that may help those of you who are struggling not only physically but emotionally. As you may know, we are not made up of only a physical being. Our beings also include a mental, emotional, and spiritual state. All four states work together for correct function. When one part of your being is not functioning optimally, then all the other parts may not be performing as well as they could be. It's like being a chair with different size legs or one missing. If the chair isn't properly built with four legs the same size, it will not be a functioning chair. Therefore, I have listed some resources (books and links) that have helped me throughout the years, and I'd like to offer them to you.

Is This Book for You?

In my opinion, it is for everyone who wants to lose body fat! Though I specialize in women's fitness, health, and weight loss, the principles in this book are meant for just about everyone:

- ✓ both male and female
- ✓ the young and the young at heart
- ✓ those with pre-menstrual syndrome (PMS), perimenopause, and menopause
- ✓ those with hypothyroidism
- ✓ those with gluten and lactose intolerances, as well as diabetes

The principles are primarily based on health, but they will also boost your performance and move you towards your goal of that youthful sexy body you so long for.

What You Must Do To Be a Success

For some, the steps given to help lose body fat and live a healthy lifestyle will be easy. But, I won't lie. For some, it will be difficult. It all depends on how you were raised and how you've been conditioned. No matter what, you've taken the right step by picking up this book. Your intention, and dedication to yourself, is a great start in helping you make some very positive changes that will benefit your health, performance, and body. You won't regret making the effort.

Sure, you may take a step backwards, but that's part of life. We all go through ups and downs. Building healthy habits take time, and you will learn how to build those habits with the pillars of health that I'm going to show you. You just can't give up. Habits built upon good principles are going to keep you healthy and trim for a lifetime. I think the biggest misconception of healthy foods is that they are bland tasting, and that is why many people take those steps backward as they miss those good tasting foods. But, don't let those misconceptions fool you. You will learn some simple techniques here that will liven up healthy foods and make you crazy for more.

As your personal coach throughout this book, I will do my best to help you along every step of the way. If you are slipping off the straight and narrow road to your success, you don't have to fall in the ditch. Before you even continue reading this book, you have a wonderful support system in place that will help you. My Facebook forum is a great place for encouragement, motivation, and accountability. Doctors and personal trainers are there to help as well. The atmosphere is very friendly, and newcomers are always a delight. There is no spam and only great help. So, please feel free to join for more support. Who knows! You may even be a voice for someone else. The group is: http://www.facebook.com/groups/BurnFatLoseWeight/. In addition, I have created another Facebook support group for just those who have questions relating to this book, *One Size Does NOT Fit All Diet Plan*. You may also see the FAQ (Frequently Asked Questions) under the *Books* tab on my website www.AbbyCampbellOnline.com.

More than anything, you have the tools to accomplish your goals and be a success. Your mind is your best and most powerful tool. Just remember that your desire plus your intentions will result in change. Blessing to You!

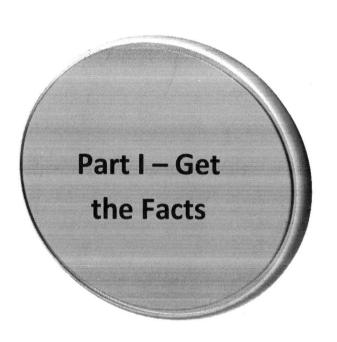

Part I – Get
the Facts

1 – The Facts on Obesity

What you will learn in this section:

✔ How one determines being overweight or obese.

✔ What causes obesity.

✔ Health problems associated with being overweight or obese.

✔ How many Americans are overweight and obese.

✔ Economic consequences of overweight and obesity.

✔ Determining if you are an individual who struggles with weight.

✔ What you can do to prevent or help your weight struggle.

How Does One Determine Being Overweight or Obese?

Both *overweight* and *obese* are labels for ranges of weight that are generally higher than what is considered healthy for a given height. The labels are also terms used to identify ranges of weight that are also related to particular health problems and diseases.[1]

On the following page is a chart that shows the ideal height and weight for both men and women. The numbers in this chart are based on the lowest calculated mortality rates for people between the ages of 25 to 59, which means that those in these weight ranges were less likely to suffer from all cause mortality than those who were lighter or heavier. Please keep in mind that body composition (i.e., muscle mass) will determine one's ideal weight.[2]

Height	Women			Men		
	Small Frame	Medium Frame	Large Frame	Small Frame	Medium Frame	Large Frame
4'10"	102-111	109-121	118-131	--	--	--
4'11"	103-113	111-123	120-134	--	--	--
5'0"	104-115	113-126	122-137	--	--	--
5'1"	106-118	115-129	125-140	--	--	--
5'2"	108-121	118-132	128-143	128-134	131-141	138-150
5'3"	111-124	121-135	131-147	130-136	133-143	140-153
5'4"	114-127	124-138	134-151	132-138	135-145	142-156
5'5"	117-130	127-141	137-155	134-140	137-148	144-160
5'6"	120-133	130-144	140-159	136-142	139-151	146-164
5'7"	123-136	133-147	143-163	138-145	142-154	149-168
5'8"	126-139	136-150	146-167	140-148	145-157	152-172
5'9"	129-142	139-153	149-170	142-151	148-160	155-176
5'10"	132-145	142-156	152-173	144-154	151-163	158-180
5'11"	135-148	145-159	155-176	146-157	154-166	161-184
6'0"	138-151	148-162	158-179	149-160	157-170	164-188
6'1"	--	--	--	152-165	160-174	168-192
6'2"	--	--	--	155-168	164-178	172-197
6'3"	--	--	--	158-172	167-182	176-202
6'4"	--	--	--	162-176	171-187	181-207

You can measure your wrist to figure whether you have a small, medium, or large frame. Wrap your right index finger and thumb around your left wrist. If your finger and thumb overlap by ¼ inch, you have a small frame. If they just touch, you have a medium frame. If they don't touch, you have a large frame.

What Causes Obesity?

There are many factors that play a role in obesity which makes it a complex health issue to address. Body weight is a result of genetics, metabolism, behavior, environment, culture, and socioeconomic status. However, being overweight or obese is mostly a result of imbalanced energy (eating too many calories + not enough exercise). Behavior and environment are the biggest culprits of this.[3]

What Health Problems are Associated with Weight?

Unfortunately, there are a host of health problems and diseases that are caused from being overweight or obese. According to the Trust for America's Health, obesity is related to more than 20 major chronic diseases.[4] Following are just a few of the increased risks identified by the United States Department of Health and Human Services agency.

> **Premature Death.** Even a little extra weight around the middle of 10 to 20 pounds increases the risk of death, particularly for those between the ages of 30 to 64. An estimated 300,000 deaths per year may be attributed to obesity in the United States.[5]

> **Heart Disease.** This includes heart attack, congestive heart failure, sudden cardiac death, angina or chest pain, and abnormal heart rhythm. One in three adults have high blood pressure, and it is twice as likely for someone who is overweight or obese compared to someone with a healthy weight.[6] An estimated one in four adults has some form of heart disease,[7] and this is the leading cause of death in the United States.[8]

> **Cancer.** Most prevalent are endometrial, colon, gall bladder, esophagus, prostate, kidney, uterine, and post-menopausal breast cancers.[9/10] Women gaining more than 20 pounds from the ages of 18 to mid-life have doubled their risk of post-menopausal breast cancer compared to those who kept their weight stable. Approximately 20 percent of cancer in women and 15 percent of cancer in men are attributable to obesity.[11] Cancer is the second leading cause of death in the United States.[12]

> **Diabetes.** A person that has gained only 11 to 18 pounds above a healthy weight has increased their risk of this disease.[13] More than 80 percent of those with type 2 diabetes are overweight or obese.[14]

Currently, there are 80 million Americans with either type 2 diabetes or are pre-diabetic.[15] Diabetes is the seventh leading cause of death in the United States and accounts for 11 percent of all health-care costs.[16]

> **Kidney Disease.** Forty percent of overweight individuals, as well as 83 percent of obese individuals, are more likely to develop kidney disease than those with healthy weights.[17]

> **Reproductive Complications.** This includes pregnancy complications such as increased death in both mother and baby, maternal high blood pressure by 10 times, gestational diabetes, high birth weight causing Cesarean section and low blood sugar, as well as increased birth defects such as spina bifida. In pre-menopausal women, there could be irregular menstrual cycles and infertility.[18]

> **Arthritis.** Those diagnosed with arthritis include 68.8 percent of overweight and obese individuals.[19]

> **Breathing Problems** Sleep apnea and asthma are common with obesity.[20]

> **Neurological and Psychiatric Diseases.** Dementia, Alzheimer's, depression, anxiety, and other mental health conditions are related to obesity. Ten research studies concluded that those who were obese at the beginning of those studies were 80 percent more likely to develop Alzheimer's disease than those who were not obese.[21] Mood disorders rose by 56 percent amongst obese individuals as well.[22]

> **Other Health Consequences.** Included are gallbladder disease, incontinence, increased surgical risk, and depression. Quality of life can be affected through limited mobility and decreased physical endurance. Children who are obese are even twice as likely to die before the age of 55 as those with healthy weight.[23]

How Many Americans are Overweight or Obese?

The United States statistics of obesity and overweight individuals has grown astronomically over the last 30 years. More than two-thirds, or 68 percent, of Americans are either overweight or obese.[24] In fact, it is the most prevalent of all countries and is the world's leader of obesity. While no state had an obesity rate above 15 percent in 1980,[25] the average obesity rate in 2008 was 34 percent[26] with more than two-thirds of states having an obesity rate above 25 percent.

The highest obesity rates, and well above 30 percent, are in the south: Alabama, Arkansas, Kentucky, Louisiana, Mississippi, Oklahoma, Tennessee, and West Virginia. Six of these 8 states also have the highest rate of hypertension, diabetes, and physical inactivity.[27]

Ethnicity and socioeconomic class seem to have a strong correlation with obesity. Blacks and Latinos have the highest obesity rates – more than Whites,[28/29] and individuals who earn 350 percent more than those within poverty levels are less likely to be obese.[30] Also, those who did not graduate high school have higher obesity rates.[31]

According to the most recent national Health and Nutrition Examination Survey (NHANES), the United States' current overweight and obesity trends in adults are as follows:[32]

> ➢ 2 of 3 adults are overweight
> ➢ 1 of 3 adults is obese

The *Journal of American Medical Association* also reports the high trend in American children for being overweight and obese.[33]

> ➢ 1 of 6 children (ages 2 to 19) is overweight
> ➢ 1 of 3 children (ages 2 to 19) is obese

These current trends show that obesity levels have increased tremendously over the last few decades. Since 1980, obesity rates have doubled for adults. Since 1970, obesity rates have quadrupled for small children (ages 6 to 11) and tripled for older children (ages 12 to 19).[34/35]

What are the Economic Consequences of Weight?

The United States has undertaken a huge hit with the economic consequences with its overweight and obesity problems. The total annual healthcare cost of obesity alone was estimated at $147 billion in 2008[36] and it is estimated to go up as high as $344 billion by 2018.[37] The majority of spending is generated from treating obesity related diseases such as diabetes which totals 11 percent of all healthcare costs.[38] Obese people spend 42 percent more on healthcare than healthy weight people.[39]

In addition to healthcare costs, obesity is costing employers approximately $4.3 billion annually just in absenteeism.[40] Lower productivity (presenteeism), medical claim costs, and indemnity claim costs also cost employers. While absenteeism alone contributes up to half of the total costs of obese employees, presenteeism costs employers $506 per year for each obese employee.[41] Medical claim costs estimate at $51,091 per 100 full-time employees compared to $7,503 per 100 healthy weight employees. For indemnity claims, costs estimate $59,178 per 100 full-time employees compared to $5,396 per 100 healthy weight employees.[42]

Are You an Individual Who Struggles with Weight?

If you are, you are not alone. With the facts already given to you, you may be shocked to find out exactly how many people are struggling with being overweight or obese. Your reach for help and hope is never too far away, and you have taken the right step by picking up this book as you will get the right guidance throughout the next several chapters.

2 – Who is Responsible for Making Society Fat?

What you will learn in this section:
- ✓ Who is responsible for making you fat.
- ✓ Why other diets have failed you.
- ✓ How most diets cause weight plateaus.
- ✓ When harsh calorie diets cause decline in metabolism.
- ✓ What choices you have and where you may go from here.

Who the USDA Is and Their Influence

The "gold standard" of nutrition education came into effect in 1992 with the United States Department of Agriculture (USDA) Food Guide Pyramid. This particular nutrition guideline has been the most widely recognized in the world while being used by most licensed doctors, nutritionists, dieticians, and other professionals dealing with nutrition education. It not only has been used by those seeking nutrition counseling. It has even been used to educate children in schools.

The original hierarchical pyramid presented itself with six food groups with daily recommendations of servings.[43]

1. Grains (breads, cereals, rice, and pastas) – 6 to 11 servings
2. Vegetables – 3 to 5 servings
3. Fruits (including fruit juices) – 2 to 4 servings
4. Proteins (meats, poultry, fish, dry beans, eggs, and nuts) – 2 to 3 servings
5. Dairy (milk, yogurt, and cheese) – 2 to 3 servings
6. Fats, oils, and sweets – use sparingly

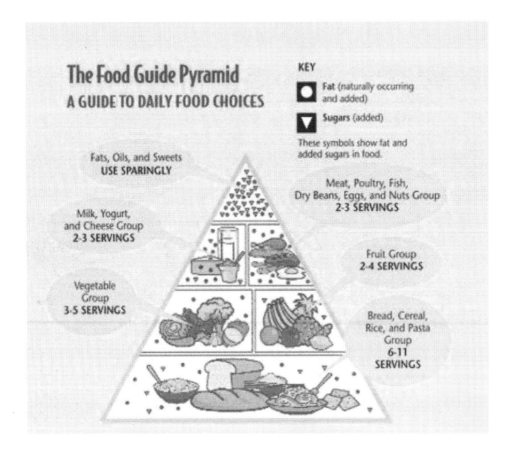

Though a nutrition guideline is a great educational tool to use for planning meals, the USDA Food Guide Pyramid of 1992 was greatly flawed. Due to its failings, its widespread adoption by nutrition professionals, consumers, and educators has contributed to an overweight and obese American society. The model included the following flaws:

➤ Grains such as breads, cereals, rice, and pastas are good and should complete the majority of your daily foods, about 6 to 11 servings.

➤ Fats are bad, no matter what type of fat and are categorized with sweets such as cookies, cake, and candy.

Since the 1992 model came about, more than 20 years of scientific research have been performed on dietary carbohydrates and fats. The results strongly support the fact that carbohydrates such as the ones that the USDA have recommended (breads, cereals, rice, and pastas) are especially not good while fats can actually be very beneficial to health. Due to the results, the USDA revised this pyramid in 2005 (called *My Pyramid*) which reflects new recommendations for its six food groups.[44]

1. Grains (now half = whole grains) – 4 servings per day (8 oz. each)
2. Vegetables – 3 cups per day
3. Fruits (now de-emphasizing fruit juices) – 2 cups per day
4. Meats and beans (includes peas, nuts, and seeds) – 6.5 ounces per day
5. Milk (includes other dairy foods) – 3 cups per day
6. Oils (now recommending fish, nut, and vegetable oils) – 7 teaspoons per day

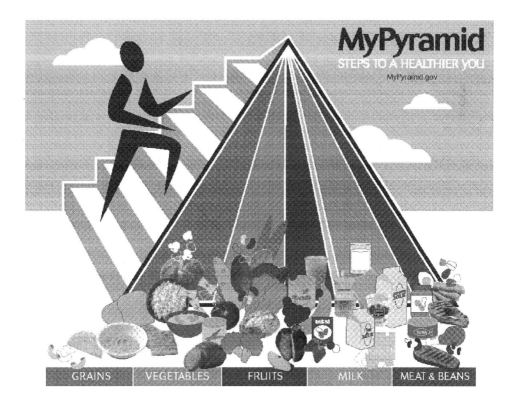

The reduction of grains and an increase of healthy fats is definitely an improvement to the original USDA Food Guide Pyramid of 1992. Improvements also included an actual volume and weight for servings. With the 1992 model, a "serving" was never defined. Therefore, it was left to the individual to decide how big or small each serving was supposed to be. Exercise was also included in the 2005 model. These are all substantial improvements to dietary advice.

In mid-2011, the USDA once again restructured the model for nutrition guidelines.[45] They replaced the triangular food pyramid with the *My Plate* model. It is a diagram of a dinner plate split into four uneven quadrants with vegetables and fruits taking up half the plate. Grains and proteins make up the other half. A cup represents the need for milk.

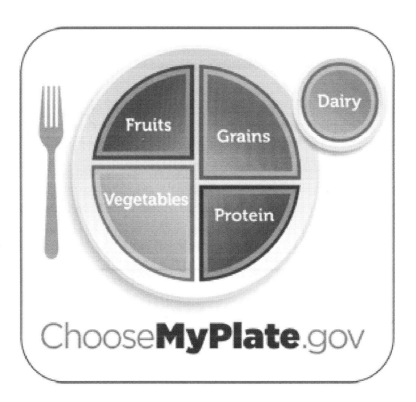

Along with the new My Plate model, the USDA even provides an interactive website for individuals to customize dietary needs. Many positive changes have taken place by the USDA through the latest nutritional guideline model and its website. However, there are still many flaws as they made a great effort to simplify the educational process of individuals wanting to eat healthier:

> **The new guideline FAILS to provide recommendations for individuals with different goals.** All people are not the same size which declares that all individuals have different body types (i.e., thin, athletic, overweight, or obese). Each of these body types responds well to different macronutrient splits (i.e., proteins, carbohydrates, and fats). However, the USDA nutrition guidelines are based on only one type of diet which consists of 15 to 20 percent protein, 50 to 55 percent carbohydrates, and 25 to 30 percent fats. These guidelines may help the individual making the switch from the typical pre-packaged, processed, and junk food diet. On the other hand, it is not the ideal for everyone as each individual has different goals. Those who are thin may have a goal of gaining weight, while those who are overweight or obese may have a goal of losing body fat. Still yet, those who are very active or athletic have other goals. Each goal requires individualization in which body stats need to be considered which may include age, gender, weight, height, body fat, hormonal status, and activity level. The USDA fails at providing this individualization.

> **The new guideline FAILS at recommending too much milk as scientific research has shown there are multiple risks associated with milk consumption.**[46] Risks include exposure to hormones, lactose intolerance, potential increase for certain types of cancers, and more. The USDA recommends a high intake of milk to ward off osteoporosis, a debilitating disease where bones lose mass and become brittle due to calcium loss. Calcium is an important mineral that strengthens bones and is found in milk and other food sources. However, research has shown that milk actually does not provide much protection against osteoporosis. Better protection can be provided through other calcium rich foods such as contained within most dark green leafy vegetables as collards, turnip greens, and kale.

> **The new guideline FAILS to educate individuals on food types within food groups.** An individual would have to learn the difference between the more nutritional foods for the body versus the less desirable ones that do not provide the body with much benefit. This may include the differences between whole grains versus highly processed grains, healthy lean meats versus unhealthy fatty meats, or Omega-3 fats that provide essential nutrients for brain health versus Omega-6 fats that may cause bodily inflammation if eaten too much. On another note, the USDA has grouped the wrong foods within each of their food categories causing much complication to the individual who has a desire to learn. For instance, they group beans, nuts, and seeds within the

protein category. Though each of these foods does have some proteins, it does not contain enough to be included within the protein category. (We will learn more about food categories in a future chapter.)

> **The new guideline FAILS to provide nutrition information relating to exercise.** For those who are sedentary or don't exercise, this may be fine. Those who are active, however, will benefit from suggestions on nutrient timing for exercise in which the USDA fails to provide.

> **The new guideline FAILS to provide information on supplementation value.** This is important when nutritious food intake is limited. It provides extra insurance to the body to perform optimally. Many benefits can be obtained through supplementation, and information is lacking on the USDA's part.

Though the USDA has made great strides and positive changes in nutrition guidelines since 1992, much damage had already been done to society. Americans had already become accustomed to the dietary principles laid out in the 1992 model. That particular generation raised their families with those guidelines, and the new generation's principles and habits have passed from generation to generation unfortunately. Nor does change come easily to a society with conflicting media messages, stores chocked full of non-nutritious processed foods, and junk foods readily available at most fast food restaurants. An overweight and obese society is the result of the damage already.

Why Most Diets Fail & "Health" Foods Cause Addiction

Are you someone who put your trust in a particular diet yet have failed after a short time? Failure may equate to weight plateaus, ability to stick to the plan, or even the inability to lose body fat. Don't feel bad. Most people have tried these same diets and experienced the same struggles. Unless you've been officially educated in the field of nutrition, you most likely placed your trust in an enticing plan that isn't really based on solid nutrition facts or dependent on science. Many authors even dangle their doctoral degrees on a book cover hoping you'll trust them all the while giving no references to back their claims. Others were overnight TV show sensations, all the while giving out conflicting nutrition advice. Who can blame them as they were made to be celebrities though only educated in areas such as cardiology, psychology, etc.? Moreover, media can be very persuasive in their advertising. Manufacturers will even stamp their own health seal of approval on their food products (whether healthy or not).

Confusion can easily be formed with all the labels on different diets as well. You've probably heard of diets based on low-carbohydrate, low-fat, high-protein, etc. Who is right? The diet craze is forever here and everywhere. These diets with their never-ending and conflicting messages have failed you. There should never be a "one-size-fits-all" dieting approach! Let's go over the two most common mythical diets briefly so that you may learn the truth of why they are the ones you want to avoid in the future.

Low-Carbohydrate Diets. Most weight loss diet plans are low-carbohydrate. They usually have a reasonable amount of protein with a high dietary fat intake. Many of these diets don't specify "healthy" protein or fat intake. They only care that you are limiting your intake of carbohydrates because they know you will most likely lose weight by sticking to their diet approach. However, limiting all carbohydrates is a dangerous game. Not only are whole grain and starchy carbohydrates limited, such as breads, cereals, and pastas. The most important foods for your body are limited. Vegetables and fruits are also carbohydrates and are necessary to your health and longevity. Vegetables and fruits provide your body with a ton of nutrients (i.e., vitamins, minerals, and phytonutrients) which help protect you from free radicals, boost your immune system, fight inflammation, and repair your cells. In other words, they help your body fight off disease such as arthritis, heart disease, and cancer.[47] Sure, you may lose weight on low-carbohydrate diets, but it's not always body fat that you'd be losing. Fast weight loss usually occurs in the first couple of weeks of low-carbohydrate diets because they deplete your body muscle and liver glycogen. Essentially, you're losing water weight. If you continue to lose weight on low-carbohydrate diets thereafter, then it's because you are consuming less energy (calories) than what you're expending.

Low-Fat Diets. Many weight loss diet plans called "low-fat" eliminate as much dietary fat as possible. It provides the notion that dietary fat makes the body fat. There is absolutely no science behind this type of logic. In fact, dietary fat is a very important energy source. In the right balance, it will actually help the body lose body fat. The body needs two essential fatty acids through dietary fat: linoleic acid (an omega-6 fatty acid) and linolenic acid (an omega-3 fatty acid). Overall health is dependent on the right balance of these fatty acids.[48] Unfortunately, dietary fats got a bad rap due to two types: saturated and trans. Saturated fats can be found in beef, coconut oil, butter, cheese, and milk. Saturated fats were once associated with diseases such as Alzheimer's, breast and prostate cancers, kidney disease, diabetes, stroke, and more. Several research studies have found this false in recent years, so we may conclude now that saturated fats don't pose a threat to health.[49] Trans fats are man-made dietary fats used in pre-packaged, processed foods to make foods taste better as well as preserve foods. These "trans" fats contribute to a host of health risks: high cholesterol levels, heart disease, Alzheimer's disease, lymphoma, and more.[50] It's in your best interest to stay away from this processed type fat for optimal health.

All in all, most diets on the market have failed you because they are not based on scientific fact. You'll learn more about this later in the book, but eliminating any of the macronutrients (i.e., protein, carbohydrates, or fats) is detrimental to your health. Not only do they cause food binges and weight plateaus, but they cause metabolism decline. Once you've been on a particular unbalanced diet, your body becomes accustomed to it. Anytime it sways from it, you are looking at rebounding to the state you were in before you started the diet. Stay away from any diet that eliminates a macronutrient or uses the one-size-fits-all approach.

> *"... manufacturers are putting certain ingredients into their products to make you not only enjoy the taste but to addict you."*

Moreover, manufacturers of food products are advertising everywhere to get your attention to buy their foods. Advertisements will entice you with television, radio, internet, mailings, coupons, in-store banners, and large bulletin boards you may see driving down the road. They are all promising you that you will be slim, beautiful, and sexy if you use their products. Unfortunately, the majority of them are lying to you. The fact of the matter is that their products will make you obese and sick. They're not going to tell you what their products are really made of because you would never buy them if you knew. Besides, how would you know exactly what is good or bad when you see the ingredient labels on these products? Certain ingredient names have been changed on product labels as a disguise for those who know these products are not healthy. You would have to carry a reference book full of ingredients just to check if a food product is healthy, and that can make for a very long shopping trip.

In lieu of advertising, manufacturers are putting certain ingredients into their products to make you not only enjoy the taste but to addict you. Why on earth would they do that? As with all business ventures, they want to keep your business for profit. Some of the most addictive ingredients they use are refined sugar, high fructose corn syrup, monosodium glutamate (MSG), and aspartame. You may even see or hear advertisements on television or radio defending some of these products. High fructose corn syrup is one of them. Let's take a brief look at why they are addictive and dangerous to your health:

> **Refined sugar and high fructose corn syrup are two of the most addictive and harmful substances you can put into your body.** In fact, new research studies show that both of these substances are even more addictive than cocaine due to its cross-tolerance and cross-dependence between it and addictive drugs. This is due to the sweet receptors you carry on your tongues and its inability to adapt to the high consumption of sugar and high fructose corn syrup in modern times. When these receptors are greatly stimulated by high intake, your brain is generated with reward signals (making you feel good) that have the potential to rescind normal self-control mechanisms. Your brain won't give your body the signal that it is satiated and it will therefore want more. This leads to addiction. Too much refined sugar or high fructose corn syrup will make you gain body fat.[51/52] Research even shows that high fructose corn syrup promotes cancer cell growth.[53]

> **MSG is another addictive food substance that is thought to be a food preservative but is actually a food flavor enhancer in mostly low-fat and non-fat foods, but is present in other foods as well.** It is also an excitotoxin or neurotoxin, a class of substances that damage and kill neuronal cells within the body, causing a degenerative effect on the brain and nervous system. MSG enters the brain through membranes in the mouth, thus entering the bloodstream as MSG foods are digested. Studies have shown that MSG induces obesity, metabolic syndrome, and type 2 diabetes. Diet will not even help with obesity when excitotoxins are present.[54/55]

"Diet will not even help with obesity when excitotoxins are present."

Reports have also shown that MSG contributes to brain cell damage and trauma, retinol degeneration, endocrine disorder, stroke, epilepsy, neuropathic pain, schizophrenia, anxiety, depression, Parkinson's disease, Alzheimer's disease, Huntington's disease, and amyotrophic lateral sclerosis.[56]

> **One of the most dangerous addictive substances is aspartame which is an artificial sweetener known better as NutraSweet, Equal, or Spoonful.** Many pre-packaged foods such as diet sodas, flavored packets for water, and diet foods are sweetened with aspartame.

Manufacturers are also continually adding aspartame to foods, such as gum and cereals, even though they are already sweetened with other types of sugars. Aspartame is made up of three chemicals: aspartic acid, phenylalanine, and methanol. Aspartate is similar to MSG in that it is an excitotoxin, crossing the blood-brain barrier and causing damage and death in cells. Aspartame combined with carbohydrates cause excessive amounts of phenylalanine in the brain. This excess can decrease serotonin levels in the brain which lead to emotional and mental disorders such as depression, anxiety, and schizophrenia. Methanol is a deadly poison. When it reaches 86 degrees Fahrenheit in temperature, it breaks down into formic acid and formaldehyde. Since the body is normally set at 98.6 degrees Fahrenheit, all living tissues are embalmed. Aspartame accounts for 75 percent of adverse reactions to food additives reported to the USDA.[57] There are over 90 different symptoms documented with migraines, muscle spasms, depression, fatigue, insomnia, heart palpitations, slurred speech, and joint pain being some of the few. According to physicians and researchers, certain diseases are caused, aggravated, or accelerated by aspartame: brain tumors, lymphoma, multiple sclerosis, fibromyalgia, epilepsy, Parkinson's disease, Alzheimer's disease, and diabetes.[58]

How Most Diets Cause Weight Plateaus

At any given moment, 25 percent of all men and 33 percent of all women are on some sort of formal diet within the United States. More than 66 percent gain back all of their weight and more than what they started with.[59] Unfortunately, most diets are a one-size-fits-all approach. With any diet book you pick off the bookstore shelf, or any old diets passed down by your great aunt, you'll find the *same* diet for everyone. Some of those are completely unsound nutritionally while others may be backed by good nutrition principles. Yet, even those with good nutrition principles don't personalize their approach to fit each person's body makeup. They are unfortunately a one-size-fits-all dieting approach.

Your body makeup signifies whether your body is thin, athletic, overweight, or obese. A person who is thin is not going to eat the same as someone who is athletic or even obese. Even with two women trying to lose weight, each would have a different approach depending on body stats. Why on earth would a woman at 120 pounds and another at 250 pounds be on the same diet and eat the same amount of calories? Sure, the 250 pound woman would lose weight to begin, just as the 120 pound woman would. However, weight loss progress declines and comes to a complete halt for the heavier woman after several weeks or a few months on the same exact diet plan. Why so? It's because she placed herself in "starvation mode."

What is starvation mode? It is when your brain thinks you are starving and goes into protection mode. Your brain doesn't know you're just trying to lose body fat. It thinks you are starving it because it's not getting enough food to support all of your body's functions. It's craving the vitamins, minerals, and phytonutrients it is lacking while in starvation mode. Wanting more so that your body and brain functions optimally, it holds onto what it does have for protection sake. It's holding onto your body fat. When your brain gives your body this signal, you stop losing weight which is called a "weight plateau."

Your body needs energy, and that energy comes from food. With too much energy, it gains weight (particularly body fat). Too little energy will cause weight loss. However, if your energy deficit is too great, then plateaus will form and you'll stop losing weight. Your body stats (i.e., age, gender, weight, height, body mass, body fat, hormonal status, and activity level) will determine how much energy you actually need. A heavier person will need more than those who are lighter in weight. An athletic person will need more than those who aren't active. Most importantly, your body requires a certain amount of energy just to sustain your body's vital functions at rest. This is called your resting metabolic rate (RMR), and it accounts for over 70 percent of your total energy. Yes, that's correct. Over 70 percent of your expended energy is required just to sustain life without movement. The heavier you are, the more energy you need to carry your weight and feed all the cells within your body. Therefore, your RMR will be higher. In the case of a 250 pound woman, she will need much more energy (calories) than a 120 pound

> *"What is starvation mode? It is when your brain thinks you are starving and goes into protection mode. Your brain doesn't know you're just trying to lose body fat. It thinks you are starving it because it's not getting enough food to support all of your body's functions."*

woman just to function and stay alive. If your body does not receive the food and nutrients it needs, it will decline. Your body will then hold onto all stores of body fat as the brain is telling it that an emergency has occurred.

A one-size-fits-all approach to dieting puts just about everyone in jeopardy of weight plateaus. Once a weight plateau occurs, losing weight becomes even more difficult.

When Harsh Calorie Diets Cause Decline in Metabolism

You've probably heard of the terms "high metabolism" and "slow metabolism." It's common for people to think that thin people have high metabolisms while overweight or obese people have slow metabolisms. However, this is rarely the case. Metabolism is usually dependent upon an individual's eating and exercise behaviors. Sure, there are some rare underlying conditions that may contribute to a slow metabolism such as hypothyroidism. Hypothyroidism, or underactive thyroid, refers to a condition in which the thyroid gland is not receiving enough of a certain hormone that is important for the normal balance of chemicals within the body.[60] Most overweight and obese people do not have underlying conditions as their weight gain is usually due to an energy imbalance (high calorie intake through food and little calorie expenditure through activity and exercise).

Since most people who opt for a calorie or fat reduction diet are those who have more than 10 to 15 pounds to lose, the one-size-fits-all type diets endanger the body's metabolism. Your metabolism refers to your biochemical processes that sustain life.[61] These processes allow you to grow, reproduce, repair damage, and respond to your environment. With part of your metabolism, two processes occur: catabolism and anabolism.

Catabolism breaks down the body by excreting energy. It provides the body energy it needs for physical activity from the cellular level on up to whole body movements. When you eat, your body breaks down the organic nutrients such as proteins, carbohydrates, and fats which release energy. Some catabolic hormones include:

> **Cortisol.** Produced by the adrenal cortex, cortisol is also known as the "stress" hormone. It raises blood pressure and blood sugar while reducing immune responses.

> **Glucagon.** Produced by the alpha cells in the pancreas, glucagon stimulates breakdown of glycogen by the liver which causes blood

sugars to increase. (Glycogen is carbohydrates stored in the liver and used for fuel during physical activity or exercise.)

> **Adrenaline.** Produced by the medulla of the adrenal gland, adrenaline is also known as the "fight or flight" reaction in response to fear. It will cause your heart to beat faster, strengthening force of heart contractions.

> **Cytokines.** Cytokines are small proteins that are released by cells of the immune system and act as mediators between cells, especially during immune response or injury. Inflammation occurs when cytokines are doing their job.

Anabolism allows your body to build new cells and maintain all tissues. Like a home contractor may use bricks and mortar as building blocks to create a home, anabolic processes use a few simple chemicals and molecules to build more complex molecules (i.e., proteins, carbohydrates, and fats) for your body. For instance, bone growth and muscle mass increase are caused by anabolic processes. Some other benefits of anabolic hormones include:

> **Bodily Growth.** Growth hormones of the pituitary gland stimulate the release of the liver hormone, which in turn causes growth.

> **Fetus Reproductive Growth.** IGF-1 and other insulin-like growth hormones activate the growth of the uterus and placenta, as well as the early growth of the fetus during pregnancy.

> **Female Reproductive Growth.** Estrogen develops female gender characteristics, strengthens bones, and regulates the menstrual cycle.

> **Male Reproductive Growth.** Testosterone develops male gender characteristics, as well as strengthens bones and muscles.

> **Sugar Regulation.** Insulin regulates sugar levels in the bloodstream.

Basically, catabolism creates the energy that anabolism consumes. If catabolism creates more energy than anabolism requires, there will be excess energy in which the body stores glycogen or body fat.

Catabolism – Anabolism = Body Weight

What Choices You Have and Where to Go From Here

A diet plan doesn't have to be as complicated as what it may seem to you. You have a choice and that is to educate yourself on good nutrition principles – principles that are based on scientific research. You've begun that by picking up this book. In the following few chapters, you will learn what those principles are.

3 – Growing Nutritionally

What you will learn in this section:

✓ Understanding a diet meal plan that is tailored to you specifically.

No matter what goals you have in life, you still need to take chronological steps to get there. A baby doesn't walk before he crawls. An 18 year old doesn't graduate high school before going through elementary and middle schools. A doctor only practices medicine after she has gone through medical school. To develop the body you want, you must also go through chronological steps.

If you were a marathoner, you would first learn the systems of exercise and institute a proper plan to reach your goal of 26.2 miles in 3.5 hours. You would have to start off with much less running distance and build your stamina over a period of time, especially if you had been living a sedentary lifestyle. Without taking the proper steps towards your marathon goal, you would mostly likely poop out before the first mile and end up quitting before you really ever got started. With a goal in place, your initial mission may be running one quarter of a mile for three days the first week. The second week, your goal may be running one half of a mile for four days. From there, you would build your distance and endurance over a period of weeks, months, or years. Eventually, you will reach your goal of 26.2 miles. You as a marathoner would also have to learn to eat a proper diet to fuel your body's system for such a strenuous goal. By picking up this book, you have taken the initial step towards your goal of losing body fat and eating for a healthy lifestyle. It is highly suggested that you learn these nutrition principles in chronological order of the phases, as those who rush towards the finish line without proper steps usually never reach their goals. For those who do reach their goals, but without the appropriate steps, usually fall backwards and become frustrated that they are back at step one again. Success usually comes with building steps in a precise manner, and your patience will help if you want to succeed for a lifetime.

Nutritional Age #1: Crawl Before You Walk

Nutrition can be very complicated if you make it that way, and this is what most people do who want to lose weight. They will pick up a one-size-fits-all diet book and do exactly what it tells them to do: clean out the refrigerator and pantry, go grocery shopping for expensive and hard-to-find foods they never heard of, and eat the exact amounts the book tells them. Some may even decide that they only need a certain amount of calories, as well as a certain amount of macronutrients (i.e., proteins, carbohydrates, and fats), all the while wracking their brains day after day with calculating numbers to lose a certain amount of weight each week. The problem with this is that they are making dieting way more difficult than it really needs to be, while a one-size-fits-all approach does not work long-term. Because of these laborious plans, many find themselves quitting within a short amount of time only to start again with a new and different plan that is really just as complicated as the time before. A vicious cycle has been put into place. The worst part is that goals become obscure and true success is never reached.

In Phase 1 of this plan, you will learn how to crawl before you walk. What does that mean? Well, you won't need any complicated meal plans to follow. You won't even have to search out every grocery store in town to find difficult foods. Best of all, you won't have to do any number crunching with calories or macronutrients. Besides, number crunching is usually for the experts so let's just leave it to them for now. What you will do is focus on building good eating habits with *real* healthy foods. You may find this to be easy as some of these healthy foods and habits have already been learned. Then again, you may take a little longer on building these healthy habits, but the principles and the process are still simple as you will see.

You will find 9 principles of healthy eating in this initial phase. To incorporate these principles into your life, you must build habits which are done over time. You've probably heard the quote, "It takes 21 days to form or break a habit." Some habits may be harder to build than others, but that's okay. If it takes you

21 days or even four months to build one good habit, then you are doing well. The days and months you spend on each habit may seem like an eternity while you are building it, but it is actually only a fraction of time when looking at the overall picture of your life. What better way to really focus and work on yourself during this time so that you can live a healthy productive life for the rest of your life! Another wonderful quote about habits reminds me of just this. It's by Doug Henning and says, "The hard must become habit. The habit must become easy. The easy must become beautiful." You may find that forming one good habit is difficult at first, but it will get easier. Once you've reached that stage, a beautiful work has been formed as you are moving closer to the healthy lifestyle you so desire.

Working on 9 principles or habits may seem like a long time with working on each for 21 days or longer. The sum is a little more than six months at 21 days each. Don't be discouraged by this! Remember that it took you much longer (maybe your whole life) to build bad habits that helped you gain weight or form illnesses. In comparison, six months is just a fraction of that time. You are worth giving that time and attention to. No one loses weight overnight.

> *"The hard must become habit. The habit must become easy. The easy must become beautiful." ~Doug Henning*

Studies have shown that permanent loss of body fat comes with building good eating habits, not from silly miracle pills and diets.[62] In addition, good eating habits don't mask the pain or symptoms of illnesses as medications do. They can be used as a prescription for healing. So, relax and enjoy this time of learning, building, and healing.

Picture your favorite sports car. After cranking the engine, imagine the nice humming sound of the exhaust. Brrrrmmmm! It only sounds that way because you treated it right by filling its tank with proper gasoline and replacing the dirty oil with clean. If you didn't do this, your beautiful baby sport won't be sporting much longer. It will become a clunker, breaking down and dying before you really even got a chance to play with it. What a shame that would be! Now picture your body as that sports car. It also needs to be filled with the right stuff (i.e., nutrients) to run optimally and live a long life. You do this by building healthy habits.

While you are building great eating habits based on these 9 principles, you will be surprised at the changes in your body, as well as your mind. A cleansing process will take place. This will start from the inside and work itself towards the exterior. You will start feeling healthier and more energetic. Then you will notice your clothes are fitting a bit looser. You'll find yourself happier than you were previously, and your outlook on life will be much brighter. What a glorious moment! If there is ever a warning in this, you may find these good habits to be addictive.

Nutrition should be simple for 90 percent of people. You may find that you never need to advance to the next stage of your nutritional age once you embrace these principles. Your body will be transformed just by building good eating habits, and simplicity is extremely nice.

Nutritional Age #2: Walk for Life

Now that you've learned to crawl, you may walk. You've built great habits and are making healthy food choices, but you may want to personalize an eating approach a bit more. There are many reasons for this. You may want to plan out your meals to stay better organized. A plan may also help you stick to your habits better. Seeing your plan day in and day out may even teach you what food combinations are appropriate. Whatever your intention, a more structured eating plan will assist you in fine tuning your goals.

Phase 2 of this nutritional plan is meal planning. The thought of planning your meals may seem quite overwhelming, but it doesn't have to be. In fact, it's quite simple with this phase. There is still no calorie or macronutrient counting. However, you will learn to get organized with your meals. Being organized will help you with grocery shopping and cooking, and it may even help you along further in your weight loss.

The majority of people may never need to go past this phase. Goals will be reached through good eating habits, and bodies will be transformed.

Nutritional Age #3: Race for the Choice

If you want to take your body to the next level, you may have super goals. You may have dreams of being a super model or accomplishing pro-level physique. Your performance goals may be of athlete status. This phase is also for those who tried Phase 2 but need more direction on serving sizes to help them move closer to their goals. Whatever your goals, you have a strong desire to take your body to the next transformation level.

Phase 3's nutrition plan is for those who have the discipline to follow with 90 percent adherence or higher. Blueprints are built for high level individualization. There is still no calorie or macronutrient counting with this plan as it has already been done for you; however, adherence is important. Depending on your specific plan, you will have blocks (servings) of particular foods already calculated. Examples are given which you may use, or you may build your own individualized plan by using the blueprints. Some minor calculations will need to be done in personalizing the plan but this is simple compared to calorie and macronutrient counting. Because you desire to take your transformation to the next level, an assumption is made that you will be including exercise. Therefore, blueprints are included for such.

You will find three parts for Phase 3 as this plan is highly individualized. You will have blueprints for days that you can use for strenuous exercise days, less stringent exercise days, and no exercise days (rest days). More calories are required for strenuous exercise days while less is required for normal exercise or cardio days. Rest days require even less calories. Calories aren't the only difference amongst the three plans though. The types of nutrients, as well as nutrient timing, are considered for each plan.

Many people may never use the blueprints of this plan, but it is provided as a comprehensive plan for all people who do want individualization to reach their goals in the shortest time possible without weight plateaus. Though Phase 3 may be a bit more complex than Phase 1 or 2, it is still a simple plan for those who need such a meticulous one.

Nurture after the Race

After running the race of Phase 3, you will need to change up your nutritional plan so that you are maintaining your goals, or your weight. You have a few choices here:

1. Go to Chapter 11 for transition and maintenance nutrition.
2. Afterward, you may go back to Phase 1 or Phase 2 for more simplified nutrition.

At this point, you will have the tools to eat healthy for life. Stick to the 9 principles of Phase 1, and you will never go backwards. You will stay fit and trim. Health will be on your side. Feeling healthy inside and out will shine forth, and you will enjoy life with much confidence.

4 – Your Desire + Intention Equals Change

What you will learn in this section:
- ✓ Planning goals and deadlines will help you stay focused.
- ✓ Self-evaluating is the initial step to making changes.
- ✓ Determining your cost of achieving or not achieving goals.
- ✓ Reading and studying is the best education for making informed food decisions as well as motivate you.
- ✓ Getting rid of stinkin' thinking by replacing thoughts with positive words will be life-affirming for you.
- ✓ Executing your plan, tracking your progress, and rewarding yourself will help you succeed.

Making up your mind is by far the most important key to building a healthy body. As mentioned in the introduction, "desire plus intention equals change." Your mind is a powerful thing. It is very important that you put your energy into focusing on things that you want to achieve and not on the things that you want to avoid or fear.

Have you ever wondered why you can't make headway with the changes you desire? Do you wonder why you keep sabotaging yourself or falling off the wagon? What about resisting those little chocolate chip temptations? You will only hinder yourself if your behavior is controlled by your subconscious mind which has accumulated negative thoughts and habits over time.

So, how do we fix the stinkin' thinking you've accrued all these years? First, you really need to focus on your conscious thoughts. Stop feeding your subconscious with negative statements. Carrying on these mental conversations need to be nipped in the bud. Some of the statements that the subconscious brings to the forefront of the conscious are:

I don't want to be fat anymore...

I wish I could get rid of this gut...

I love food so this will never work...

My parents gave me the fat gene...

I'll try, but...

I don't have time to workout...

I have a slow metabolism...

I hate being fat!!!!!!

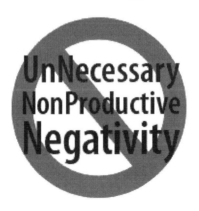

You have control over 100 percent of your thoughts, so you must master your communication with yourself. You must overwrite your stinkin' thinking! Replace those old negative thoughts with positive ones that will help you achieve. Before you know it, your subconscious mind will only be speaking good things to you, and you will have reached your goals. Replace some of those negative statements with these life-affirming statements:

I'm not going to be fat anymore!

I'm going to enjoy the process of losing body fat!

I'm going to learn to love healthy foods!

I'm totally responsible for my results!

I'm going to do this no matter what it takes!

Working out every morning makes me feel alive!

My metabolism is getting faster by the day!

I love my body!!!!!!!!!

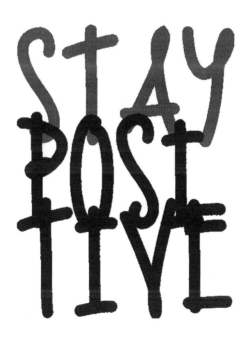

Switching your mind from negative thoughts to positive ones is not going to be easy. After all, negative thoughts do turn into habits. In order to change, you will need to evaluate and set some goals for yourself. You may initiate the following 9 steps to get started:

Step #1 - Self-Evaluate

Review your behaviors that have held you back from achieving your goals. Try to list five current behaviors that are preventing you from fulfilling your goals. With each behavior, write down your new behavior that will allow you to accomplish your goals. See the self-evaluation example below. The form may be found in the Appendix of this book.

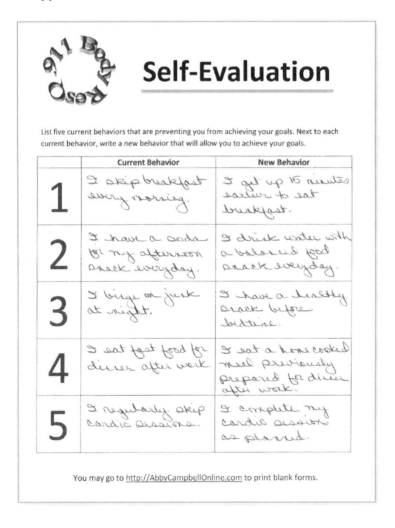

Step #2 - Plan Goals

What are your top five fat loss, fitness, and health goals? With each goal, list two behaviors that you can do to move towards achieving each goal. An example has been included below, and the form may be found in the Appendix of this book.

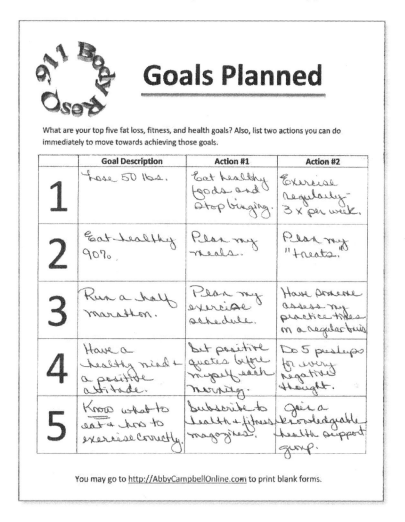

Goals Planned

What are your top five fat loss, fitness, and health goals? Also, list two actions you can do immediately to move towards achieving those goals.

	Goal Description	Action #1	Action #2
1	Lose 50 lbs.	Eat healthy foods and stop binging.	Exercise regularly - 3 x per week.
2	Eat healthy 90%.	Plan my meals.	Plan my "treats."
3	Run a half marathon.	Plan my exercise schedule.	Have someone assess my practice times on a regular basis
4	Have a healthy mind + a positive attitude.	Set positive quotes before myself each morning.	Do 5 pushups for every negative thought.
5	Know what to eat + how to exercise correctly.	Subscribe to health + fitness magazines.	Join a knowledgable health support group.

You may go to http://AbbyCampbellOnline.com to print blank forms.

Step #3 - Plan Deadlines

Set realistic deadlines for the five goals you planned in Step 2. Make an "overall" deadline to complete all your goals. A form has been provided for you in the Appendix called "Goal Deadlines."

Step #4 – Evaluate Goals

Placing a value on your goals will help you see what you will gain or lose by achieving or not achieving your goals. This gives real perspective to what you really want. Evaluate your goals by answering the following four questions. A form has been included in the Appendix.

1. What is the cost of achieving your goals?
2. What is the cost of NOT achieving your goals?
3. What will you experience if you succeed in your goals?
4. What will you NOT experience if you do NOT succeed in your goals?

Step #5 – Read and Study

Reading enriches the mind, and what better way to learn as much as you can on how to achieve your goals! Broaden your knowledge base through reputable magazines, books, internet articles, and forums. The more you have the information drilled in your head, the more motivated you will be. A recommended reading list is also included after the Appendix at the end of this book.

Step #6 – Be Positive

Encourage yourself by being positive. Tell yourself that you will achieve your goals and forget about the stinkin' thinking. When you start feeding yourself positive thoughts, a chemical reaction occurs in your brain and you start seeing things a bit differently. You won't be stressed as much, and you'll have more energy to do the things you love. You will even start appreciating the little things more. If it helps, place positive quotes in areas that you will see every day to motivate yourself. See the next page for some popular quotes that may help you as you set out on a new healthy lifestyle path.

Surround yourself with positive people who will help you succeed. By hanging out with people who share similar goals or at least support you will help you achieve your goals much easier. You also have a free support group you can join right now at https://www.facebook.com/groups/BurnFatLoseWeight/.

"If I find 10,000 ways something won't work, I haven't failed. I am not discouraged, because every wrong attempt discarded is another step forward. Just because something doesn't do what you planned it to do doesn't mean it's useless."

~Thomas Edison

"All I have is today. All I have is this moment, this workout, this meal, the next 30 minutes, the next hour. If I just do what I know I must do now, then I know I'll reach my ultimate goal eventually."

~Tom Venuto (Natural Bodybuilder)

"I can do all things through Christ who strengthens me."

~Philippians 4:13

"Mistakes are natural. Mistakes are how we learn. When we stop making mistakes, we stop learning and growing. But repeating the same mistake over and over is not continuous learning – it's not paying attention."

~Wally "Famous" Amos

Just Do It!

Step #7 – Work It

As Nike would say, it's time to just do it! Your plans and goals are in place. You are ready to execute the plan. It's time to pay close attention to your planner every single day. Spend a few minutes early in the morning going over your schedule for the day. Reread your goals. Get motivated with your favorite quotes. Then ask yourself, "What time will I be exercising today?" and stick to the schedule. Make a mental note of when your meals are scheduled, and just stick to the plan. What do you have to pack for lunch? What do you need to take out of the freezer to thaw for dinner? Get your mind together so that you know what needs to be done. Gear up for the day! If you do what you know you're supposed to do, you will succeed. So, JUST DO IT!

Step #8 – Track Progress

You've already executed the plan and have been doing so for a while now. It may be a week or even a month. Even though your pants may be a little looser or you feel much healthier after applying the 9 principles of healthy eating, you may want to track progress in a more formal manner. Tracking your progress will show you exactly what changes you have made and how much closer you are to your goal. There are several ways that you can track your progress. Some of the best ways of tracking are as follows:

1. Weekly weight check (with a reliable body weight scale)
2. Monthly girth measurements (with a reliable cloth measuring tape)
3. Body fat measurements (only if you can with a personal trainer & calipers)
4. Monthly or quarterly pictures (full front, side, and back views)

By tracking your progress, you will determine whether you need to tweak your plans. If you're making changes, there is no need to change anything unless you want to. If you're not making changes, then you need to review your actions since you started the plan. Be honest with yourself. If you haven't been adhering to the plan at least 90 percent of the time, then you need to tighten up. If you are adhering to the plan completely and still aren't seeing changes, then it's time to modify it with either your meals or exercises.

Tracking forms, as well as measurement forms, that may help you with your progress are located in the Appendix.

Step #9 – Reward Yourself

Whenever you reach one of your goals, reward yourself. You can either have a meal that you really miss after reaching a certain weight or inches lost. (Of course, don't go hog wild and eat a whole pizza and a half tub of ice cream!) However, rewards don't have to be food. A professional massage or pedicure could be your reward. What about those spunky shoes you've been eyeballing at your favorite dress boutique or men's store? You may even want to predetermine your "big" rewards for your "big" goals when you are in the planning stage. A fun-filled shopping spree for a whole new wardrobe could be an exciting "big" reward. Maybe a day at the spa? Or, you can go real big and get that new sporty car that you've had your heart set on for the last five years! Whatever your heart's desire, let that be your motivation!

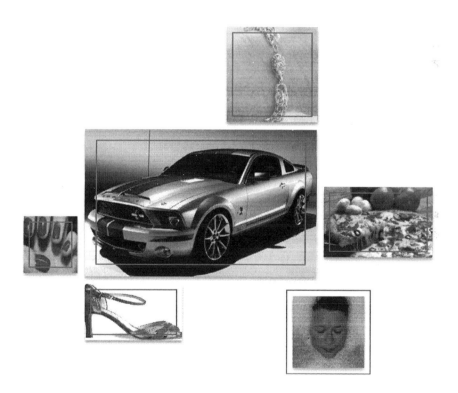

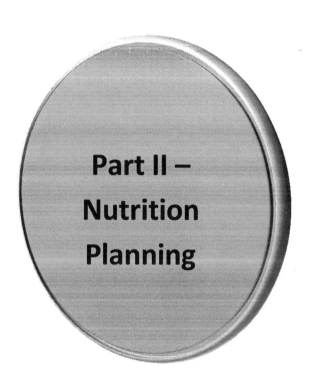

Part II –
Nutrition
Planning

5 – Phase 1: SMART EATS

What you will learn in this section:
- ✓ **S**upplying you with nutrients at regular intervals.
- ✓ **M**aking natural foods a part of your lifestyle.
- ✓ **A**cquiring enough protein with each meal and snack.
- ✓ **R**eaching for vegetables and fruits at every meal.
- ✓ **T**aking in starches for after workouts only.
- ✓ **E**mbracing healthy fats.
- ✓ **A**cquiring only water and herbal teas for beverages.
- ✓ **T**reating you with weekly rewards.
- ✓ **S**implifying meal preparations.

Phase 1 nutrition planning is for those who have not mastered healthy eating. In other words, if you are just beginning your journey of living healthy and are learning what healthy foods are, this phase is for you. It is also for those who do know what healthy eating principles are but may need a refresher course to get back on track. By mastering this phase, you will have built habits in using all 9 principles on a regular basis without really thinking about them. Until you do master this phase, it is unnecessary to move to Phase 2 or 3, though Phase 2 may help you stay more organized after understanding the 9 principles.

There is no calorie counting in this phase. The goal is for you to learn new healthy habits by mastering these 9 principles – The SMART EATS principles. Just know that you will see changes in your body. You will see changes as quickly as the first week when you come from a background of unhealthy pre-packaged, processed, and refined foods. Your body will make changes from the inside out. At first, you may begin feeling healthier, more vivacious, and full of energy. Losing weight (body fat) is just a nice side effect.

Why is there no calorie counting? Calorie counting for most is burdensome, including those who are in the profession of fitness and nutrition. It takes time to plan and track calories. Besides, it's not all about calories when it comes to a healthy and balanced diet. To plan correctly, you must also track macronutrients such as protein, carbohydrates, and fats. If you don't do this correctly, then you may be harming yourself more than helping. Now talk about burdensome! Many fail at dieting because they feel the need to track calories and then end up quitting because they learn that it's not only difficult, but they also don't have the time and energy for it. As babies must learn to crawl before walking, so must you who are learning to eat healthier. You must first learn to eat the right foods before you can jump into being on the level of a nutritionist. By learning to eat the correct foods in the right balance, you will lose weight and get healthy. The SMART EATS principles will show you how to do this naturally. You may even find that you will never have the need to go any further in planning. Most people will do best in Phase 1 of nutrition planning. They will lose body fat just by eating the right foods in the right ways. No need for technical number crunching!

For some of you, these 9 SMART EATS principles will be easy to grasp and you will be well on your way. For others who have grown up to a completely different eating approach, you will have to alter your lifelong habits and it may be difficult at times. If you find these habits are difficult to build, take it one step at a time. Focus on one principle at a time for however long it takes to grasp (it doesn't have to be in the order given here either). Each principle may take two weeks or two months to build. That's perfectly fine. You have to give yourself a break as it took a lifetime to build your current habits. Though the time you take may seem like forever to grasp a new habit, it is miniscule compared to the lifetime of habits you already have. Remember, these 9 principles are setting you up for the remainder of your life – a healthy life. What's two weeks or two months in the process if you need that time? Let's get started, but please check out Chapter 13 for preparation tips for success.

Principle #1 – Keep the Sugar Monster Away by Eating at Regular Intervals

"I see food, I eat food." This is the mentality of most people and is what has made an overweight and obese society. Research has shown that eating at regular intervals, every two to four waking hours, is important for not only health but for body composition as well. Some health benefits from using this strategy are:

➤ **Balanced blood sugar.** Skipping breakfast and eating once or twice per day can lead to a physiologic response that promotes fat storage.[63] By eating at regular intervals, every two to four hours, your body stabilizes blood sugar levels. By avoiding insulin spikes, you will be avoiding weight gain.[64]

➤ **Less cravings and overeating.** By eating every two to four hours, you will have less cravings and less chance of overeating.[65] Overeating causes insulin spikes which will make you gain body fat.

➤ **Better mental and physical performance.** Brain fog sets in when the body is craving nutrients. You may be able to focus and perform better throughout the day when you nourish your body and brain with foods at regular intervals.[66]

➤ **Metabolism boost.** Eating every two to four hours tells your brain that it's going to continually receive nutrients. It therefore signals your body to digest and assimilate those calories and nutrients faster knowing that more food is to come. A faster metabolism burns more body fat.[67]

➤ **Muscle preservation.** By not getting the nutrients at regular feedings, lean muscle mass catabolizes (breaks down).[68] You want to preserve lean muscle mass as it burns body fat.

Total Meals Per Day = Time Awake ÷ 3 Hours	**What if I'm not hungry?** Then skip your meal and try to eat less at your next meal.	**Meal size?** Do not overstuff yourself. Eat until you are 80% full.
3 meals & 2 snacks? Sure, as long as all "feeding opportunities" are nutritionally balanced.	**Missed meal?** No worries. Just get back on track & try to do better the next day.	**Bedtime meal?** Yes, if your mealtime falls within that time frame.

Principle #2 – Eat Natural Foods: Calories Worth Their Weight in Gold

A calorie is a measure of energy. Energy status in the body, or body weight change, depends on energy intake versus energy expenditure. Energy intake is made up of the calories taken in by the foods you eat. Energy expenditure includes physical activity, vital function at rest, digestion of foods, and bodily waste. If energy intake is greater than the output, body weight is gained. If energy expenditure is greater than the input, body weight is lost. If energy intake and expenditure are equal, body weight is maintained. One pound of body fat stores 3,500 calories. To lose that one pound of body fat, energy will need to burn the same amount of calories (3,500).

You've probably heard that a calorie is just a calorie and all that matters in losing weight is dependent on how many calories you are taking into your body. Though this is true to an extent, there are many other factors to be considered. The types of food you put into your body also matter:

➢ **Natural foods burn more energy than processed foods.** Natural foods are made from the earth, animals, and fish. This includes foods such as vegetables, fruits, whole grains, tubers, legumes, lean beef, poultry, eggs, and fish. Processed foods are commercially prepared foods for convenience. They are usually foods that have been altered or preserved in packages, boxes, jars, cans, or plastic such as frozen dinners, white bread, and boxed cookies. They also have a long shelf life. Research shows that whole foods consume nearly 50 percent more energy when digested than the *empty* calories provided by processed foods.[69]

➢ **Fiber foods reduce calorie absorption.** Fiber is a form of carbohydrates found in vegetables, fruits, whole grains, tubers, and legumes. They contribute to satiety (feeling full) but their calories don't count because they are not absorbed into the body. High fiber foods are also calorically dense and have less dietary fat and sugar.[70]

➢ **Protein foods burn more calories than carbohydrates and fats.** The thermic effect of food increases energy expenditure that comes from the digestion and processing of nutrients in food. A specific dynamic action occurs between protein, carbohydrates, and fats. Research has shown that protein boosts metabolism by 20 to 30 percent while carbohydrates boost metabolism by five to 10 percent and fats zero to five percent.[71] For every 100 calories you ingest, 20 to 30 calories will be burned for digestion and absorption while leaving a net of 70 calories for protein.

Principle #3 – Melt Body Fat Like Crazy with Proteins

Protein is a very important nutritional building block, especially for body composition. For optimal health, you should have protein at every meal and snack. Some quality protein foods to include in your diet include lean beef, skinless chicken breast, turkey, pork tenderloin, seafood, fish, and egg whites. If you don't have a lactose or dairy intolerance, low-fat cottage cheese, Greek yogurt, and skim milk are also great sources. Some great non-animal sources of protein include tofu and tempeh. Quality isolate protein powders are also great sources, especially post workout or as a supplement when in a time crunch.

Protein is needed for many reasons. It keeps your blood's PH levels balanced, maintains proper hormone levels, and regulates proper fluid balance. It preserves muscle (especially in times of dieting) and is an energy source when there are no carbohydrates available. Your immune system relies on protein for proper functioning.[72] Protein is also very beneficial for weight loss:

➤ **Higher metabolic rate**. Protein is thermogenic and leads to increased metabolism. It burns at least twice as many calories as carbohydrates and fats, which provides you with greater fat loss. When protein is overeaten, gaining fat is difficult.[73]

➤ **Increased glucagon**. Protein increases glucagon which is a hormone that fights the effects of insulin. Unregulated insulin levels will wreak havoc on the body leading to potentially severe health problems. Glucagon also helps decrease the making and storing of body fat, which also means higher fat loss during dieting and less fat gain while overeating.[74]

➤ **Growth hormone regulation**. Eating enough protein ensures your body is getting all amino acids which are the building blocks to make growth hormones. Metabolism is slowed if you don't get enough growth hormones, which can lead to lower bone density, muscle loss, and a number of other physiological and mental issues.[75/76]

➤ **Increased IGF-1**. Protein increases IGF-1 which is an anabolic hormone that increases muscle growth. Higher IGF-1 spares muscle while dieting, and it increases muscle mass while overeating.[77]

➤ **Anabolism**. Eating protein keeps your body in an anabolic, or constructive, state. Not getting enough protein causes muscle catabolism or deterioration. Muscle tissue burns body fat, so keeping your body in an anabolic state is important for weight loss.[78]

See Chapter 12 for healthy protein foods.

Principle #4 – Love Your Vegetables & Fruits

You may be someone who hates vegetables and/or fruits with a passion and therefore are cringing with just the thought of this type of food, but have you really given them a chance? There are tons to be taste tested, and many can be prepared in a variety of ways. You just need to find what suits you.

Vegetables are the absolute best source of carbohydrates as they provide a plethora of nutrients and antioxidants that you can't get from other food types. By consuming a diet high in vegetables and fruits, you are lowering your risk for chronic diseases such as cancer and cardiovascular disease.[79/80] Most days, they will provide your body with enough glucose for a healthy body. In addition, vegetables and fruits will help you lose weight for a variety of reasons:

- ➢ **Fewer calories provide fat loss.** Because vegetables and fruits are lower in calories, you can eat more and get more satiated than if you were eating foods higher in calories. Studies show comparisons of eating vegetables and fruits with eating high calorie processed foods. To get full on each, the amount of calories coming from vegetables and fruits was half that compared to the high calorie foods.[81]

- ➢ **Increased water and fiber provide fullness.** Vegetables and fruits have a high water and fiber content. The impact of water adds weight to these foods without increasing calories.[82] Whole fruit has even proven to have a higher satiety than pureed or juiced versions of the same fruit.[83] Numerous studies have shown that high fiber diets result in weight loss.[84]

- ➢ **Fiber eliminates waste.** Fiber in vegetables and fruits provide healthy bowel function as it keeps food moving through the digestive tract and providing quicker elimination. This gives a boost in overall gut health and also reduces fat and cholesterol in the bloodstream.[85]

- ➢ **Fiber is indigestible.** Fiber is the indigestible part of plant sourced foods such as vegetables and fruits. Your body cannot digest or absorb fiber. Therefore, fiber calories are not processed.[86]

- ➢ **Blood sugar is stabilized.** Vegetables, and fruits in the right serving sizes, have a low glycemic index. While high glycemic index foods raise blood sugar levels quickly, low glycemic foods sustain blood sugar levels and insulin concentrations which in turn enhance satiety, energy level, and body composition.[87]

See Chapter 12 for all healthy carbohydrate choices.

Principle #5 – Meet Starchy Foods after the Gym Only

Starches are carbohydrates like vegetables and fruits. Though some are nutritious, they still don't provide your body with the mega vitamins and nutrients that vegetables and fruits do. In fact, they are usually loaded with calories, even for small amounts. Starchy carbohydrates include whole grains, tubers, and legumes. They also include foods such as pasta, cereal, bread, and snacks like cake, cookies, and potato chips. However, the foods mentioned in the last sentence are refined and highly processed. Natural starches such as oats, quinoa, brown or wild rice, sweet potatoes, and beans are much healthier choices.

Unfortunately, refined carbohydrates have become a dietary staple in the American culture, as well as most western cultures, and have contributed to many chronic diseases such as coronary heart disease, diabetes, and cancer.[88/89/90] Though research shows that whole grains protect against coronary heart disease, other studies have shown that whole grains may also contribute to insulin sensitivity and type 2 diabetes, especially if eaten in excess.[91/92] Recent studies have also shown that all starchy carbohydrates (especially the refined type) are likely to cause metabolic health damage to those who are predominantly sedentary and overweight.[93] This is most likely due to the overeating of these foods. Does that mean that whole grains are off limits? Not necessarily, but our plan does eliminate whole grains that contain gluten (i.e., wheat, rye, and barley) as recent research has shown that these foods are currently causing havoc on physical and mental health due to being genetically modified.[94/95] However, you know your body best, so judge for yourself on whether gluten foods are a hindrance to your weight loss efforts.

Nutrient timing of natural starchy carbohydrates is very important. Starchy carbohydrates mostly benefit those who exercise on a regular basis, and especially *after* a strenuous workout for those who want to lose body fat.[96/97] Starchy carbohydrates are best utilized after a strenuous workout to help your body recover faster. After strenuous exercise such as cycling and weight training, muscle energy stores are depleted and need to be replaced. By including starchy carbohydrates within the first two hours after exercise, muscle damage has been reduced while recovery has been improved.[98/99] Your brain and central nervous system require a continuous supply of glucose.[100] When it is too low, your muscles catabolize. If it is too high, it will turn to body fat. It is very easy to over-eat starchy carbohydrates, and this is why it is only recommended post workout. At other times, you will get vegetables and fruits, as carbohydrates in all forms are essential to life.

Principle #6 – Don't Allow Fat to Be Your Enemy

Contrary to what you've been told, dietary fat is not your enemy. The "No Fat" or "Low Fat" diet is a diet of the past, though there is some legitimacy to those concepts. During those fads, more and more people were opting for fast foods, as well as pre-packaged, processed, and refined foods. These foods contained "trans" or "hydrogenated" fats which are chemically processed and unnatural fats used to preserve foods.[101] Many health risks are a result of these unnatural fats such as cardiovascular disease, Alzheimer's disease, and cancer.[102/103/104] Recent research has even proven that trans fats contribute to irritability and aggression.[105] Fortunately in recent years, the USDA ruled a mandatory declaration in nutrition labeling of trans fats present in foods and supplements for consumer review.[106]

Natural dietary fats are an important energy source; in the formation of your cell membranes, brain, and nervous system; in the balance of hormones; in the promotion of a healthy immune system; and to keep inflammation low.[107] However, all natural dietary fats are not created equal but are equally important to your body. There are three main categories of natural fats: saturated, monounsaturated, and polyunsaturated. All three categories are thus broken down into sub-categories. For overall health, it is important for you to get a combination of all three major categories of dietary fat.

> *"Dietary fat is your friend – not your enemy!"*

However, focusing on foods that have proven to be the healthiest of all dietary fats can boost your health. Omega-3 fatty acids come from the polyunsaturated category of fats and include cold water fish such as salmon, mackerel, halibut, sardines, tuna, and herring. Other great Omega-3 food sources include scallops, shrimp, tofu, flaxseed, flaxseed oil, chia seeds, and walnuts. Research has shown that Omega-3 fatty acids can heal and prevent heart disease, high cholesterol, high blood pressure, diabetes, cancer, rheumatoid arthritis, osteoporosis, pre-menstrual cramps, macular degeneration, and mental disorders and diseases.[108] In addition, Omega-3 fatty acids have been proven to help with weight loss by improving insulin sensitivity and using stored body fat for energy.[109/110]

See Chapter 12 for healthy dietary fat choices.

Principle #7 – Get Drunk with Water & Teas

Do you drink beverages that contain calories? Beverages such as sodas and fruit juices contain a good amount of calories that usually come from sugar. Some sodas may have zero calories but are still processed and contain addicting substances such as high fructose corn syrup and aspartame. One of the best things you can do for your health, as well as for your weight loss goals, is to get rid of these types of beverages from your diet. Instead, stick to water, teas, and coffees. In fact, water and green tea are likely the beverages that will give you the best benefits.

> *"Water is your secret weapon in losing weight."*

Your body is made up of nearly 60 percent of your total body weight. That's a lot of water! Of course, how much water you carry is dependent upon your body fat, muscle mass, and levels of hydration. Different cells within your body contain different amounts of water: 22 percent in bones, 25 percent in body fat, 75 percent in muscles, and 83 percent in blood. As you can now see, water is essential for your entire body. In fact, water benefits your body in a variety of ways. It carries nutrients and oxygen to cells, protects body organs, regulates body temperature, lubricates joints, moistens mucous membranes, helps the kidneys and liver by flushing out waste products, and helps prevent constipation.[111] Recent studies have also shown that water is your secret weapon in losing weight. Just by drinking two cups of water prior to each meal helps you lose more weight than if you didn't drink those two cups.[112]

Tea and some coffee beverages have been shown through research to benefit your body in numerous ways. This is possibly due to the polyphenols, natural chemicals classified as being antioxidants, anti-viral, and anti-inflammatory properties. Polyphenols protect your body from free radicals that cause damage. Green tea is especially beneficial as it has been shown to prevent and inhibit cancer growth; protect against cardiovascular disease, diabetes, and DNA damage; and boost immunity.[113/114] Abundant studies have shown that green tea plays a role in decreasing body fat by increasing energy expenditure and fat oxidation.[115]

Adding water, teas, and coffees to your daily menu plan will help reduce your urge for sugar-filled beverages. By including at least 8 cups of water and two to three cups of herbal tea throughout the day, you will find that you are satiated longer. You may also find that you feel slimmer. Better than that, you will be slimmer!

Principle #8 – Have a Treat: Stick to the 90/10 Rule

Are you one of those people who does "all or nothing" when it comes to things in life? Maybe you've even tried this approach with dieting in the past only to find failure. Studies show that when dieters feel deprived, they are more likely to binge on forbidden foods and end up quitting. In fact, this is one of the top reasons why most diets fail.[116] Binging on foods that you know you're not supposed to makes you feel like a cheater. Well, this plan eliminates the word "cheat" when it comes to dieting. Cheaters are scammers, deceivers, and defrauders. Cheating only conjures up feelings of guilt and remorse which is unnecessary when you are working your tail off trying to get healthier.

Instead, this plan is going to allow you have a "treat." A treat is a goody, a pleasure, and a celebration. You deserve a treat when you're working so hard! Just because you are creating good healthy habits of eating does not mean you have to give up on foods you have always loved that may not be considered healthy. Instead of trying to fool everyone by sneaking around to eat something you know you shouldn't have, you are going to reward yourself. Besides, you can't fool anyone! After all, you would only be deceiving yourself. Right? If you enjoy traditional pizza, spaghetti, and Chinese food, reserving them as treats is a

> *"... reward yourself the other 10 percent of the time."*

way to still include them as part of your diet plan. Just don't overdo it! Celebrating your week of hard work with one or two slices of pepperoni pizza and a side salad is much more sensible than having a whole pizza!

How often are you allowed to have treats? If you promise to watch your quantities, you're allowed to have goodies 10 percent of the time. In other words, stick to the healthy eating principles laid out in this chapter 90 percent of the time and reward yourself the other 10 percent of the time. If you eat four meals per day (this includes snacks), that is 28 meals per week when you multiply by seven days. Ten percent of 28 meals equates to two to three meals per week. Remember that keeping your treats within proportion and not overdoing it is the key if you want to make progress towards your weight loss and health goals. If you're a stickler about being "all or nothing," I challenge you to include this rule. Many fitness experts have used this strategy with their clients to only find success.[117]

Principle #9 – Gain a New Favorite Hobby in Cooking

Let's face it! We live busy lives, and the days of preparing gourmet meals are a bygone. Most people just don't have the time for it. Everyone wants quick and easy! You will need some tasty and easy meals with variety that you can make day in and day out. Planning your meals is the best way to staying on track. Just make sure you are sticking to the 8 previous healthy eating rules on a consistent basis.

Planning? You probably thought there wouldn't be any with this first phase of meal planning. Well, you may not be laying out every single meal for the week, but you still need to plan to go grocery shopping and have the right foods available. If you don't at least plan to have healthy options in your refrigerator and pantry, then you're only creating disaster for yourself and won't succeed towards your goals of weight loss or a healthy body.

Never cooked? It's okay. You will find very simple recipes for all types of foods in Chapter 13. In fact, they are so simple that you will wonder why you never cooked before. By using some of these recipes, you might not even have to cook every night as you can prepare foods in bulk to make your entire week easier. Don't even let the word "bulk" scare you as you will see how easy this

> *"Cooking is at once child's play and adult joy. And cooking done with care is an act of love."* ~Craig Claiborne

is. Just let grocery shopping and cooking be your new hobby at least once per week, and you will wonder why you ever made healthy eating such a chore!

6 – Phase 2: Building Healthy Plates

What you will learn in this section:
- ✓ Planning and organizing healthy balanced meals.
- ✓ Using nutrient timing to further your goals.

If you have reached this phase of nutrition planning, then congratulations are in order! However, you may be surprised to hear that you do not even need to graduate to Phase 2 if you've been succeeding with Phase 1. By succeeding in Phase 1, you will not have only mastered the 9 principles of healthy eating. You will have started feeling healthier and even lost some weight and inches. If you are continually doing well with this in Phase 1, then don't fix what's not broken. Continue in Phase 1 as it's the simplest way to reach your transformation goals.

If you have mastered, or need a little more organization with Phase 1, continue with Phase 2 nutrition planning. Phase 2 will help you plan out your meals and keep you a bit more organized. Again, there is no calorie counting in this phase. Instead, you will learn how to balance meals with protein, carbohydrates, and fats. You will also better learn nutrient timing skills for certain foods to help you lose body fat. By planning your meals with Phase 2, as well as sticking to the 9 principles of healthy eating, you should get results in as little as a few days.

Below you will find simple blueprints for creating healthy balanced meals that will help you burn body fat. You may use the meal charts in Chapter 12 to help you hand-pick foods you enjoy to build your own personalized meal plan. After building a few plans, future plans will be a cinch. You may then rotate the plans you have already created or build new ones. Please see the appendix for planning forms. (For maintenance plans, see Chapter 11.)

Fat Loss Plan for Non-Workout Days

Following is a blueprint for non-workout or rest days. Even if you have a casual walk or stroll through the park, this is the plan to be used. There is no fruit or starchy carbohydrate to be eaten on this day no matter the number of meals that you need for the day. This will help eliminate the extra sugars that fruit, lentils, whole grains, and tubers contribute. In turn, you will burn body fat faster. You may find the blueprint in the Appendix.

Fat Loss Plan: Non-Workout Days
(This is a sample 6-meal menu plan)

Meal	Protein	Veggie	Fat
Meal 1 – Breakfast	eggs & turkey sausage	sautéed onions & bell peppers	(included in egg yolks)
Meal 2 – AM Snack	low-fat cottage cheese	cherry tomatoes	sunflower seeds
Meal 3 – Lunch	chicken breast	Romaine, cucumbers, onions, tomatoes (salad)	2 Tbs. natural salad dressing
Meal 4 – PM Snack	protein shake	celery & carrot sticks	natural peanut butter
Meal 5 – Dinner	grilled salmon	broccoli flowerets	Parmesan cheese
Meal 6 – Bedtime Snack	Greek yogurt	cucumber slices	chia seeds

Fat Loss Plan for Normal Workout & Cardio Days

On normal workout and cardio days, you may add in one or two servings of fruit as this will give your body the extra energy it has depleted from exercise. Fruits are placed with your post workout meal in the sample below. However, you may place it at whichever meal you like. You will find blueprints in the Appendix, and you may place your post-workout meal where it is necessary for you personally.

Fat Loss Plan: Normal Workout & Cardio Days
(This is a 5 meals sample menu plan)

Meal	Protein	Veggie	Fruit	Fat
Meal 1 – Breakfast	scrambled eggs & salmon	asparagus	NONE	(included in egg yolks)
Meal 2 – Post Workout	whey protein shake	(optional)	apple	NONE
Meal 3 – Late Lunch	turkey burger	broccoli		butter (for broccoli)
Meal 4 – Dinner	flank steak	asparagus	NONE	coconut oil (for asparagus)
Meal 5 – Bedtime Snack	hard-boiled eggs	red bell pepper slices		(included in egg yolks)

"Certain carbohydrates fuel your body with glucose more than others, with vegetables having the least and fruits and starches having the most. To maximize loss of body fat, you're going to tap into that body fat with nutrient timing."

Fat Loss Plan for Strenuous Workout Days

Fruits and starchy carbohydrates are allowed on strenuous workout days. Strenuous workout days may include heavy weight lifting, cycling, or heavy labor. You may have both types of carbohydrates, in addition to vegetables, twice per week. This will refuel your muscle glycogen and renew your energy. When you have starchy carbohydrate meals, you should eliminate dietary fat such as laid out in the post workout meal sample below. Your fruit is added to another meal of your choice. Please find blueprints for your use in the Appendix.

Fat Loss Plan: Strenuous Workout Days *(This is a 6 meals sample menu plan.)*					
Meal	**Protein**	**Veggie**	**Fruit**	**Starch**	**Fat**
Meal 1 – Breakfast	eggs & steak	spinach	*NONE*	*NONE*	*(included in egg yolks)*
Meal 2 – AM Snack	natural deli chicken slices	5 baby carrots			slice of Provolone cheese
Meal 3 – Lunch	grilled chicken breast	large salad			2 Tbs. natural salad dressing
Meal 4 – PM Snack	chocolate protein shake	**(optional)**	apple		walnuts
Meal 5 - Post Workout Dinner	tilapia fish	broccoli flowerets	*NONE*	sweet potato	*NONE*
Meal 6 – Bedtime Snack	chocolate protein pudding	greens supplement		*NONE*	flaxseed (mixed into pudding)

By sticking to the 9 principles of healthy eating and using these blueprints, you should see progress towards your weight loss goals. If for some reason you are not seeing progress, and you are including five to seven hours of exercise per week, you may (1) reduce your food portions, or (2) use the detailed meal plans which can be found in Phase 3 (Chapters 7-10) for more individualization.

7 – Phase 3: Precision Meal Planning

What you will learn in this section:

- ✓ Using detailed blueprints to build personalized meal plans.
- ✓ Learning how to use specific formulas targeted for specific needs.
- ✓ Knowing which kitchen tools are necessary for success.

Phase 3 nutrition planning is for those who have mastered the 9 principles of healthy eating, as well as for those still working on the 9 principles but need a more detailed plan to help guide them further. You will only need approximately 30 minutes to initially study over each of the blueprints for rest and active recovery days, normal workout days (includes cardio), and strenuous weight training days (or other heavy labor days). By spending about 10 to 15 minutes each morning planning out your meals, you will have a week's worth of meals by the seventh day. You can then rotate the plans you've created for future weeks. If you want 14 days of plans to rotate, then spend a few minutes for 14 days creating plans. Most of the work with planning will be in the beginning of the phase. Planning becomes easier the more you do it, and you will become accustomed to balancing meals. Eventually, meal planning for a day will only take you five minutes. After following your personalized plans for a while, you will have memorized how much each serving should contain. Before you know it, you will be a pro at meal planning.

How to Use Phase 3 Blueprints

Phase 3 blueprints for nutrition planning are broken up into three different components. Each component is for different types of activity days. Some days, you will be more active than others. Each component is targeted to fuel you for your needs for that particular day. By adjusting calories and macronutrients (i.e., protein, carbohydrates, and fats) to the type of day you have, you will prevent your body from holding weight plateaus. This type of menu planning is called "calorie/carb" cycling and the three components of this nutrition plan include:

1. Blueprints & Examples for Rest & Active Recovery Days
2. Blueprints & Examples for Normal Workout & Cardio Days
3. Blueprints & Examples for Strenuous Weight Training Days

As you can see, two components are for those who exercise. If your goal is to lose weight and obtain a healthy lifestyle, you will include exercise into your daily regimen. However, if you are not able to exercise for whatever reason, then use the first component (Blueprints & Examples for Rest & Active Recovery Days) for six days of the week and then include the third component (Blueprints & Examples for Strenuous Weight Training Days) at the end of the week. Even though you won't be exercising, you will still need to refuel your body, as well as trick it so that it doesn't adapt to the first component. Please don't skip the third component at the end of the week as you don't want to hit any weight loss plateaus. With that being said, you should include some exercise even if it's only five minutes per day to start. The easiest way for most non-active people to get started is just by taking a walk. Build on that. Before you know it, you will be walking 30, 45, or 60 minutes. In the process, you will have lost weight from both exercise and your new nutrition plan. Exercising will then become easier and easier as you'll have more energy for activities.

Count Blocks of Food Rather than Calories

You will never have to count calories by using Phase 3 even with it being so detailed and personalized. All the calorie and macronutrient counting has already been done for you. Each of the three menu components are broken down into body weight from 120 pounds to 280 pounds. As mentioned earlier in the book, a one-size-fits-all diet approach is not a personalized approach and weight plateaus are sure to occur. A 280 pound woman has different needs than a 120 pound woman and therefore should personalize her plan accordingly. If you are in-between sizes, then go with the lower weight category. For instance, if you are 236 pounds, go with the 230 pound plan. If you are more than 280 pounds, you may do one of two things. You may try the 280 pounds plan or contact http://www.911BodyRescue.com or Abby@911BodyResQ for a more personalized plan.

Each weight plan will show you the number of blocks for each category of food: protein, vegetable, fruit, starch, and fat. Below is an example blueprint for a 130 pound person on a strenuous workout day who is trying to lose weight:

Macro	Meal 1	Meal 2	Meal 3	Meal 4	Meal 5	Total
5 Meals Menu Plan – 130 lbs. *(for strenuous workout day)*						
Protein	3	3	3	4	3	16
Veggie	1	1	1	1 ½	0	4 ½
Fruit	0	0	0	0	1	1
Starch	0	0	2 ½	0	0	2 ½
Fat	2	1	0	2	1 ½	6 ½

With the shaded column for Meal 1, you will see the following number of blocks for this meal:

➢ Protein (3)
➢ Veggie (1)
➢ Fruit (0)
➢ Starch (0)
➢ Fat (2)

You would then look at the meal charts in Chapter 12 to see what each block consists of. For protein, you need three blocks of protein for Meal 1. Go to the "Protein Choices" section of the meal charts. By picking grilled chicken, you will see that one block of protein is one ounce. You will then multiply one ounce with three protein blocks as designated on your personal weight plan. You will then figure your personal serving for protein is three ounces. Please see the top of the next page as an example.

Protein Choices

Beef (lean) - 1 oz.
- Examples: flank steak, ground (95%), round steaks & tips, sirloin, roast

Bison - 1 oz.
- Examples: rib eye, round, roast, sirloin

Chicken - 1 oz.
- Examples: canned (no broth, low-sodium), breast, gizzards, liver

TOTAL PROTEIN SERVING = BLOCK NUMBER x SERVING SIZE
3 oz. grilled chicken breast = 3 blocks x 1 oz. chicken

~~~

You will then do the same for each of the other food categories (i.e., veggie, fruit, starch, and fat). By multiplying one block of veggie with your "Vegetable Choices" in the meal charts, you will find your serving size. If you want cooked broccoli, your serving size is ½ cup. If you want cooked Brussels sprouts, your serving size is ½ cup.

Vegetable Choices

Vegetable	Qty	Vegetable	Qty
Artichokes, cooked	1	Okra, cooked	¾ cup
Asparagus, cooked	8 spears	Onions, cooked	¼ cup
Asparagus, raw	5 spears	Onion, raw	½ cup
Beets, cooked	½ cup	Pumpkin, cooked	⅔ cup
Broccoli, cooked	½ cup	Radishes, sliced	1-½ cups
Broccoli flowerets, raw	1-½ cups	Sweet Peppers, cooked	½ cup
Brussels Sprouts, cooked	½ cup	Sweet Peppers, raw	1 cup

TOTAL VEGGIE SERVING = BLOCK NUMBER x SERVING SIZE
½ cup broccoli = 1 block x ½ cup broccoli

With the 130 pound meal plan example on page 69, there are zero blocks for fruit and starch. Therefore, you won't be calculating any servings for those particular foods for Meal 1. You have two blocks for dietary fats. If you check the "Essential Fat Choices" in the meal charts, you may select one teaspoon of butter and one tablespoon of slivered almonds. The butter and almonds can be mixed with the green beans for a nice vegetable dish.

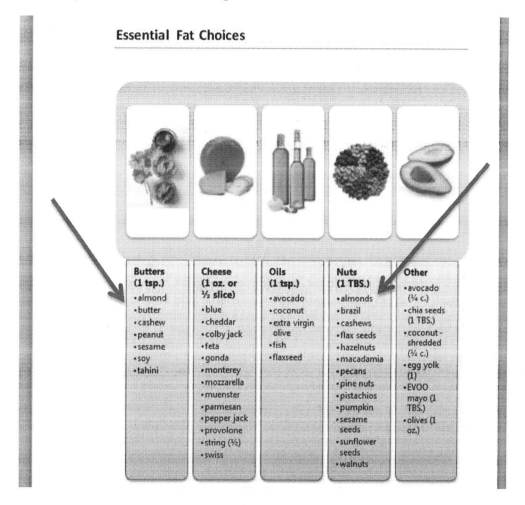

Essential Fat Choices

Butters (1 tsp.)	Cheese (1 oz. or ½ slice)	Oils (1 tsp.)	Nuts (1 TBS.)	Other
• almond	• blue	• avocado	• almonds	• avocado (¼ c.)
• butter	• cheddar	• coconut	• brazil	• chia seeds (1 TBS.)
• cashew	• colby jack	• extra virgin olive	• cashews	• coconut - shredded (¼ c.)
• peanut	• feta	• fish	• flax seeds	• egg yolk (1)
• sesame	• gonda	• flaxseed	• hazelnuts	• EVOO mayo (1 TBS.)
• soy	• monterey		• macadamia	• olives (1 oz.)
• tahini	• mozzarella		• pecans	
	• muenster		• pine nuts	
	• parmesan		• pistachios	
	• pepper jack		• pumpkin	
	• provolone		• sesame seeds	
	• string (½)		• sunflower seeds	
	• swiss		• walnuts	

TOTAL FAT SERVING = BLOCK NUMBER x SERVING SIZE
1 tsp. butter & 1 Tbs. slivered almonds = 2 blocks

~~~

To simplify, your menu would look like the following:

> ➤ Protein = 3 oz. grilled chicken breast
> ➤ Veggie = ½ cup cooked broccoli
> ➤ Fat = 1 tsp. butter & 1 Tbs. slivered almonds (mixed with broccoli)

Making Changes to Your New Weight

As you drop weight, you will need to adjust your personal menu plans with new blueprints. Dropping approximately 10 pounds, will tell you it's time. Let's say you started on your new 230 pound nutrition plan when you were 236 pounds. If you dropped down to 224 to 226 pounds, you need to move to the next weight category which is 220 pounds. This will help you from plateauing in weight and ensure that the body fat keeps melting off.

Get Your Kitchen Measuring Devices Out

Because Phase 3 is a detailed nutrition plan with particular food blocks measuring certain ounces, cups, teaspoons, etc., you will need to invest in some kitchen utensils if you don't already have them. The list is basic, and you can pick these utensils up at Wal-Mart, K-Mart, or other department stores. You may even be able to obtain these items from discount stores or EBay. Make sure you have the following:

> Digital kitchen scale that can measure ounces and grams.
> Measuring cups (measuring ¼, ⅓, ½, and 1 cup).
> Measuring spoons (measuring ⅛ tsp., ¼ tsp., ½ tsp., 1 tsp., ½ Tbs., and 1 Tbs.)

How Much Protein You Need

Though your calories and macronutrients have already been configured for this weight loss plan, some of you may be curious about how much protein you will be eating. The USDA recommends 10 to 35 percent of your total daily calories come from protein.[118] Your new nutrition plan is a cycling plan for calories, carbohydrates, and fats. However, your protein will always be the same because your needs will never change for the amount you need unless you lose or gain weight. Your protein intake will be 1.2 grams per pound of body weight which makes the percentage per day fluctuate depending on which diet component you will be using for the day. Some days will be approximately 30 percent while others may be upward of 50 percent. These amounts take you beyond the *survival* recommendations of the USDA and into the *optimal* amounts for health, maintaining muscle tissue, and losing body fat. Research has proven that including a higher amount of protein in the diet while spread evenly throughout the day shows 100 percent thermogenesis.[119] Studies have also shown that muscle loss is great when adequate amounts of protein aren't taken in while on a calorie deficit diet.[120/121]   You won't have to worry about this as you will be taking in enough protein where you will maintain muscle while losing body fat. Please review all the benefits of protein from Principle number 3 in Chapter 5.

How Carbohydrates are Calculated

Carbohydrates include vegetables, fruits, and starches, and they will be cycled depending on the diet component you are using for the day. Certain carbohydrates fuel your body with glucose more than others, with vegetables having the least and fruits and starches having the most. To maximize loss of body fat, you're going to tap into that body fat with nutrient timing. You will be using carbohydrates to fuel your body during higher activity and exercise. During other times of the day, you will allow your body access to use stored body fat as energy. By allowing your body to burn stored body fat as fuel, you will be protecting your muscle.[122]

On rest and activity recovery days, you will be eating a variety of vegetable carbohydrates which are low calorie but dense in nutrients. On normal or cardio days, you will need a bit more energy so fruits will be added to your vegetable intake. Though fruits are still pretty low in calories, they will still add a bit more energy with vitamins, minerals, and phytonutrients to help you recover from your daily exercise. Starchy carbohydrates will be added to vegetables and fruits on two strenuous workout or labor days. Because you will deplete the most energy during strenuous workouts, your body will need to re-feed. Starchy carbohydrates are calorie dense and will also replace that energy with new glycogen. This will keep you from losing energy and help you with metabolic function.[123] Carbohydrates make up approximately 10 to 30 percent of your calories depending on which diet component you are using.

How Dietary Fats are Calculated

Dietary fats make up the remainder of calories. Please review principle number 6 in Chapter 5 – Don't Allow Fat to Be Your Enemy. Dietary fat is extremely important. You want your body to burn fat. This is done by getting in enough dietary fat while reducing high calorie carbohydrates.[124]

8 – Blueprints & Examples for Rest & Active Recovery Days

What are rest and activity recovery days?

✓ Both rest and active recovery days include any days that you are not participating in activities such as weight training, kickboxing, hiking, high intensity interval training, or cardio workouts.

✓ Rest days allow your body to relax from all heavy activities during the rest of the week in order to refresh yourself, as well as allow your body to recover from the stresses placed upon it.

✓ Active recovery days allow you to be active such as with house cleaning, mowing the lawn, or taking walks, as long as it is any activity that won't raise your heart rate much for an extended timeframe.

When to Use this Blueprint

One or two rest and active recovery days should be allowed each week, especially if you have a laborious job or are doing weight training and cardio workouts on a regular basis. This allows your body to heal and recover from the stresses placed upon it during cardio and weight training days. Include the rest and active recovery blueprints for these days. Those who are also sedentary may use this blueprint for more days.

What Foods this Blueprint Includes

In order to allow your body to burn fat on rest and activity recovery days, it will include just enough calories to do so. Proteins are included to nourish your body, keep you satiated, preserve lean muscle mass, and keep your metabolism on fire. Vegetable carbohydrates are built in to supply your body with vitamins, minerals, and phytonutrients. Vegetables will also protect your body from damaging free radicals by providing it with antioxidants, and the fiber in vegetables will help rid your body of metabolic waste. Dietary fats, combined with proteins and vegetable carbohydrates, will balance out your meals and will help supply you with essential nutrients for every cell in your body to function optimally. Fruit, lentil, whole grain, and tuber carbohydrates are eliminated as your body will not need the sugars or starches during rest and activity recovery days.

How to Count Blocks of Food

An example of counting blocks of food has been given in the previous chapter. However, a new example detailing this particular blueprint has been given below.

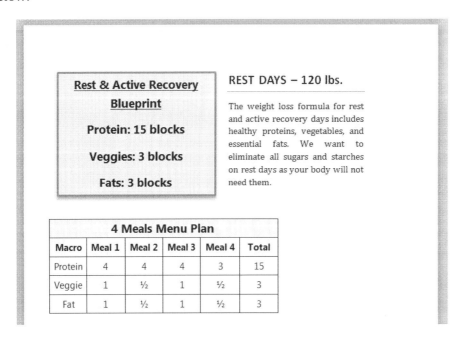

Rest & Active Recovery Blueprint

Protein: 15 blocks

Veggies: 3 blocks

Fats: 3 blocks

REST DAYS – 120 lbs.

The weight loss formula for rest and active recovery days includes healthy proteins, vegetables, and essential fats. We want to eliminate all sugars and starches on rest days as your body will not need them.

4 Meals Menu Plan					
Macro	Meal 1	Meal 2	Meal 3	Meal 4	Total
Protein	4	4	4	3	15
Veggie	1	½	1	½	3
Fat	1	½	1	½	3

For this component of Phase 3 nutrition planning, you have the option of choosing from four, five, or six meals per day. The example just given shows the "4 Meals Menu Plan." At the top of each page, you will see the blocks of food allotted for this weight category. There are 15 protein blocks, 3 veggie blocks, and 3 fat blocks for the "4 Meals Menu Plan" of the 120 pound menu plan. On the opposite page, you will be given examples for each menu plan as shown below.

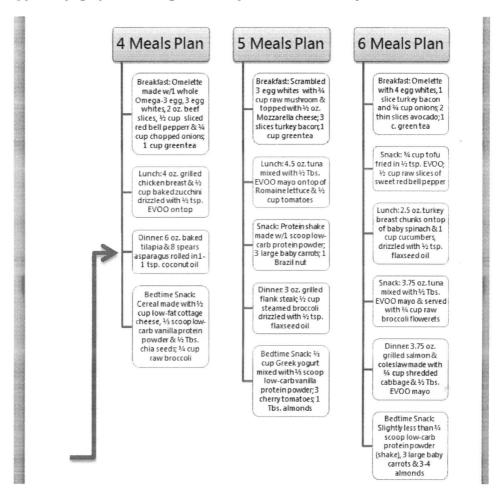

On the 120 pound menu plan, you will see how many blocks are allotted for each meal. Look at Meal 3. It includes 4 protein blocks, 1 veggie block, and 1 fat block. If you then look at the dinner meals example for the "4 Meals Menu Plan" above, you will see that that it consists of six ounces of baked tilapia (4 proteins), 8 spears of asparagus (1 veggie), and one teaspoon of coconut oil (1 fat). The foods selected are taken from the meal charts in Chapter 12 to find the serving size of each food by using the block number given on the menu plan multiplied by the serving size given on the meal charts. You may refer to the previous chapter to determine correct calculations.

Rest & Active Recovery Blueprint

Protein: 15 blocks

Veggies: 3 blocks

Fats: 3 blocks

REST DAYS – 120 lbs.

The weight loss formula for rest and active recovery days includes healthy proteins, vegetables, and essential fats. We want to eliminate all sugars and starches on rest days as your body will not need them.

4 Meals Menu Plan

Macro	Meal 1	Meal 2	Meal 3	Meal 4	Total
Protein	4	4	4	3	15
Veggie	1	½	1	½	3
Fat	1	½	1	½	3

5 Meals Menu Plan

Macro	Meal 1	Meal 2	Meal 3	Meal 4	Meal 5	Total
Protein	3	3	3	3	3	15
Veggie	½	½	½	1	½	3
Fat	½	½	½	½	1	3

6 Meals Menu Plan

Macro	Meal 1	Meal 2	Meal 3	Meal 4	Meal 5	Meal 6	Total
Protein	2 ½	2 ½	2 ½	2 ½	2 ½	2 ½	15
Veggie	½	½	½	½	½	½	3
Fat	½	½	½	½	½	½	3

Following are example menus for the weight loss formula covering rest and active recovery days for those in the 120 pound category. You may look at the Meal Chart to pick different foods that suit your taste buds.

Example Menus

Rest & Recovery Days

120 lbs.

4 Meals Plan

Breakfast: Omelette made w/1 whole Omega-3 egg, 3 egg whites, 2 oz. beef slices, ½ cup sliced red bell pepperr & ¼ cup chopped onions; 1 cup green tea

Lunch: 4 oz. grilled chicken breast & ½ cup baked zucchini drizzled with ½ tsp. EVOO on top

Dinner: 6 oz. baked tilapia & 8 spears asparagus rolled in 1-1 tsp. coconut oil

Bedtime Snack: Cereal made with ½ cup low-fat cottage cheese, ⅓ scoop low-carb vanilla protein powder & ½ Tbs. chia seeds; ¾ cup raw broccoli

5 Meals Plan

Breakfast: Scrambled 3 egg whites with ¾ cup raw mushroom & topped with ½ oz. Mozzarella cheese; 3 slices turkey bacon; 1 cup green tea

Lunch: 4.5 oz. tuna mixed with ½ Tbs. EVOO mayo on top of Romaine lettuce & ½ cup tomatoes

Snack: Protein shake made w/1 scoop low-carb protein powder; 3 large baby carrots; 1 Brazil nut

Dinner: 3 oz. grilled flank steak; ½ cup steamed broccoli drizzled with ½ tsp. flaxseed oil

Bedtime Snack: ⅔ cup Greek yogurt mixed with ⅓ scoop low-carb vanilla protein powder; 3 cherry tomatoes; 1 Tbs. almonds

6 Meals Plan

Breakfast: Omelette with 4 egg whites, 1 slice turkey bacon and ¼ cup onions; 2 thin slices avocado; 1 c. green tea

Snack: ¾ cup tofu fried in ½ tsp. EVOO; ½ cup raw slices of sweet red bell pepper

Lunch: 2.5 oz. turkey breast chunks on top of baby spinach & 1 cup cucumbers, drizzled with ½ tsp. flaxseed oil

Snack: 3.75 oz. tuna mixed with ½ Tbs. EVOO mayo & served with ¾ cup raw broccoli flowerets

Dinner: 3.75 oz. grilled salmon & coleslaw made with ¾ cup shredded cabbage & ½ Tbs. EVOO mayo

Bedtime Snack: Slightly less than ¾ scoop low-carb protein powder (shake), 3 large baby carrots & 3-4 almonds

Rest & Active Recovery Blueprint

Protein: 16 blocks

Veggies: 3.5 blocks

Fats: 3.5 blocks

REST DAYS – 130 lbs.

The weight loss formula for rest and active recovery days includes healthy proteins, vegetables, and essential fats. We want to eliminate all sugars and starches on rest days as your body will not need them.

4 Meals Menu Plan

Macro	Meal 1	Meal 2	Meal 3	Meal 4	Total
Protein	4	4	4	4	16
Veggie	1	½	1	1	3 ½
Fat	1	½	1	1	3 ½

5 Meals Menu Plan

Macro	Meal 1	Meal 2	Meal 3	Meal 4	Meal 5	Total
Protein	3	3	3	4	3	16
Veggie	½	1	½	1	½	3 ½
Fat	½	½	½	1	1	3 ½

6 Meals Menu Plan

Macro	Meal 1	Meal 2	Meal 3	Meal 4	Meal 5	Meal 6	Total
Protein	3	2 ½	2 ½	2 ½	3	2 ½	16
Veggie	½	½	½	½	1	½	3 ½
Fat	½	½	½	½	½	1	3 ½

Following are example menus for the weight loss formula covering rest and active recovery days for those in the 130 pound category. You may look at the Meal Chart to pick different foods that suit your taste buds.

Example Menus

Rest & Recovery Days

130 lbs.

4 Meals Plan

Breakfast: Omelette made w/1 whole Omega-3 egg, 3 egg whites, 2 oz. beef slices, ½ cup sliced red bell pepper & ¼ cup chopped onions; 1 cup green tea

Lunch: 4 oz. grilled chicken breast & ½ cup baked zucchini drizzled with ½ tsp. EVOO on top

Dinner: 6 oz. baked tilapia & 8 spears asparagus rolled in 1-1 tsp. coconut oil

Bedtime Snack: Cereal made with ½ cup low-fat cottage cheese, ⅔ scoop low-carb vanilla protein powder & 1 Tbs. chia seeds; ¾ cup raw broccoli & 3 large baby carrots

5 Meals Plan

Breakfast: Scrambled 3 egg whites with ¾ cup raw mushroom & topped with ½ oz. Mozzarella cheese; 3 slices turkey bacon; 1 cup green tea

Lunch: 4.5 oz. tuna mixed with ½ Tbs. EVOO mayo on top of Romaine lettuce, ½ cup tomatoes & 1 cup sliced cucumbers

Snack: Protein shake made w/1 scoop low-carb protein powder; 3 large baby carrots; 1 Brazil nut

Dinner: 4 oz. grilled flank steak; ½ cup steamed broccoli drizzled with 1 tsp. flaxseed oil

Bedtime Snack: ⅔ cup Greek yogurt mixed with ⅓ scoop low-carb vanilla protein powder; 3 cherry tomatoes; 1 Tbs. almonds

6 Meals Plan

Breakfast: Omelette made 4 egg whites, 2 slices turkey bacon and ¼ cup onions; 2 thin slices avocado; 1 c. green tea

Snack: ¾ cup tofu fried in ½ tsp. EVOO & ½ cup raw slices of sweet red bell pepper

Lunch: 2.5 oz. turkey breast chunks served on top of baby spinach & 1 cup cucumbers, drizzled w/½ tsp. flaxseed oil

Snack: 3.75 oz. tuna mixed with ½ Tbs. EVOO mayo & served with ¾ cup raw broccoli flowerets

Dinner: 4.5 oz. grilled salmon & coleslaw made with ¾ cup shredded cabbage, 1 small carrot stick & ½ Tbs. EVOO mayo

Bedtime Snack: Slightly less than ¾ scoop low-carb protein powder (shake), 3 large baby carrots & 7 almonds

Rest & Active Recovery Blueprint

Protein: 17.5 blocks

Veggies: 4 blocks

Fats: 4 blocks

REST DAYS – 140 lbs.

The weight loss formula for rest and active recovery days includes healthy proteins, vegetables, and essential fats. We want to eliminate all sugars and starches on rest days as your body will not need them.

4 Meals Menu Plan

Macro	Meal 1	Meal 2	Meal 3	Meal 4	Total
Protein	4 ½	4	5	4	17 ½
Veggie	1	1	1	1	4
Fat	1	1	1	1	4

5 Meals Menu Plan

Macro	Meal 1	Meal 2	Meal 3	Meal 4	Meal 5	Total
Protein	3	4 ½	3	4	3	17 ½
Veggie	1	1	½	1	½	4
Fat	1	½	½	1	1	4

6 Meals Menu Plan

Macro	Meal 1	Meal 2	Meal 3	Meal 4	Meal 5	Meal 6	Total
Protein	3	2 ½	3	3	3	3	17 ½
Veggie	½	½	1	½	1	½	4
Fat	½	½	½	½	1	1	4

Following are example menus for the weight loss formula covering rest and active recovery days for those in the 140 pound category. You may look at the Meal Chart to pick different foods that suit your taste buds.

Example Menus

Rest & Recovery Days

140 lbs.

4 Meals Plan

Breakfast: Omelette made w/1 whole Omega-3 egg, 3 egg whites, 2.5 oz. beef slices, ½ cup sliced red bell pepper & ¼ cup chopped onions; 1 cup green tea

Lunch: 4 oz. grilled chicken breast & ½ cup baked zucchini & 3 cherry tomatoes drizzled with 1 tsp. EVOO on top

Dinner: 7.5 oz. baked tilapia & 8 spears asparagus rolled in 1-1 tsp. coconut oil

Bedtime Snack: Cereal made with ½ cup low-fat cottage cheese, ⅔ scoop low-carb vanilla protein powder, and 1 Tbs. chia seeds; ¾ cup raw broccoli & 3 large baby carrots

5 Meals Plan

Breakfast: Scrambled 3 egg whites with ¾ cup raw mushroom and ¼ cup chopped onions & topped with 1 oz. Mozzarella cheese; 3 slices turkey bacon; 1 cup green tea

Lunch: 6.75 oz. tuna mixed with ½ Tbs. EVOO mayo on top of Romaine lettuce, ½ cup tomatoes & 1 cup sliced cucumbers

Snack: Protein shake made w/1 scoop low-carb protein powder; 3 large baby carrots; 1 Brazil nut

Dinner: 4 oz. grilled flank steak; ½ cup steamed broccoli drizzled with 1 tsp. flaxseed oil

Bedtime Snack: ⅔ cup Greek yogurt mixed with ⅓ scoop low-carb vanilla protein powder; 3 cherry tomatoes; 1 Tbs. almonds

6 Meals Plan

Breakfast: Omelette with 4 egg whites, 2 slices turkey bacon and ¼ cup onions; 2 thin slices avocado; 1 c. green tea

Snack: ¾ cup tofu fried in ½ tsp. EVOO; ½ cup raw slices of sweet red bell pepper

Lunch: 3 oz. turkey breast chunks served on top of baby spinach & 6 cherry tomatoes drizzled w/½ tsp. flaxseed oil

Snack: 4.5 oz. tuna mixed with ½ Tbs. EVOO mayo & served with ¾ cup raw broccoli flowerets

Dinner: 4.5 oz. grilled salmon & coleslaw made with ¾ cup shredded cabbage, 1 small carrot stick & 1 Tbs. EVOO mayo

Bedtime Snack: 1 scoop low-carb protein powder (shake), 3 large baby carrots & 7 almonds

Rest & Active Recovery Blueprint

Protein: 19 blocks

Veggies: 4 blocks

Fats: 4 blocks

REST DAYS – 150 lbs.

The weight loss formula for rest and active recovery days includes healthy proteins, vegetables, and essential fats. We want to eliminate all sugars and starches on rest days as your body will not need them.

4 Meals Menu Plan

Macro	Meal 1	Meal 2	Meal 3	Meal 4	Total
Protein	5	4	5	5	19
Veggie	1	1	1	1	4
Fat	1	1	1	1	4

5 Meals Menu Plan

Macro	Meal 1	Meal 2	Meal 3	Meal 4	Meal 5	Total
Protein	3 ½	4 ½	3	4	4	19
Veggie	1	1	½	1	½	4
Fat	1	½	½	1	1	4

6 Meals Menu Plan

Macro	Meal 1	Meal 2	Meal 3	Meal 4	Meal 5	Meal 6	Total
Protein	3	3	3	3	4	3	19
Veggie	½	½	1	½	1	½	4
Fat	½	½	½	½	1	1	4

Following are example menus for the weight loss formula covering rest and active recovery days for those in the 150 pound category. You may look at the Meal Chart to pick different foods that suit your taste buds.

Example Menus

Rest & Recovery Days

150 lbs.

4 Meals Plan

Breakfast: Omelette made w/1 whole Omega-3 egg, 3 egg whites, 3 oz. beef slices, ½ cup sliced red bell pepper & ¼ cup chopped onions; 1 cup green tea

Lunch: 4 oz. grilled chicken breast & ½ cup baked zucchini & 6 cherry tomatoes drizzled with 1 tsp. EVOO on top

Dinner: 7.5 oz. baked tilapia & 8 spears asparagus rolled in 1-1 tsp. coconut oil

Bedtime Snack: Cereal made with ½ cup low-fat cottage cheese, 1 scoop low-carb vanilla protein powder, and 1 Tbs. chia seeds; ¾ cup raw broccoli & 3 large baby carrots

5 Meals Plan

Breakfast: Scrambled 3 egg whites with ¾ cup raw mushroom and ¼ cup chopped onions & topped with 1 oz. Mozzarella cheese; 4 slices turkey bacon; 1 cup green tea

Lunch: 6.75 oz. tuna mixed with ½ Tbs. EVOO mayo on top of Romaine lettuce, ½ cup tomatoes & 1 cup sliced cucumbers

Snack: Protein shake made w/1 scoop low-carb protein powder; 3 large baby carrots; 1 Brazil nut

Dinner: 4 oz. grilled flank steak; ½ cup steamed broccoli drizzled with 1 tsp. flaxseed oil

Bedtime Snack: ⅔ cup Greek yogurt mixed with ⅔ scoop low-carb vanilla protein powder; 3 cherry tomatoes; 1 Tbs. almonds

6 Meals Plan

Breakfast: Omelette with 4 egg whites, 2 slices turkey bacon and ¼ cup onions; 2 thin slices avocado; 1 c. green tea

Snack: 1 cup tofu fried in ½ tsp. EVOO; ½ cup raw slices of sweet red bell pepper

Lunch: 3 oz. turkey breast chunks served on top of baby spinach & 6 cherry tomatoes drizzled w/½ tsp. flaxseed oil

Snack: 4.5 oz. tuna mixed with ½ Tbs. EVOO mayo & served with ¾ cup raw broccoli flowerets

Dinner: 6 oz. grilled salmon & coleslaw made with ¾ cup shredded cabbage, 1 small carrot stick & 1 Tbs. EVOO mayo

Bedtime Snack: 1 scoop low-carb protein powder (shake), 3 large baby carrots & 7 almonds

<table>
<tr><td colspan="2">

Rest & Active Recovery Blueprint

Protein: 20 blocks

Veggies: 4.5 blocks

Fats: 4.5 blocks

</td></tr>
</table>

REST DAYS – 160 lbs.

The weight loss formula for rest and active recovery days includes healthy proteins, vegetables, and essential fats. We want to eliminate all sugars and starches on rest days as your body will not need them.

4 Meals Menu Plan

Macro	Meal 1	Meal 2	Meal 3	Meal 4	Total
Protein	5	5	5	5	20
Veggie	1	1	1 ½	1	4 ½
Fat	1	1	1	1 ½	4 ½

5 Meals Menu Plan

Macro	Meal 1	Meal 2	Meal 3	Meal 4	Meal 5	Total
Protein	4 ½	4 ½	3	4	4	20
Veggie	1	1	1	1	½	4 ½
Fat	1	½	1	1	1	4 ½

6 Meals Menu Plan

Macro	Meal 1	Meal 2	Meal 3	Meal 4	Meal 5	Meal 6	Total
Protein	3	3	4	3	4	3	20
Veggie	1	½	1	½	1	½	4 ½
Fat	1	½	½	½	1	1	4 ½

Following are example menus for the weight loss formula covering rest and active recovery days for those in the 160 pound category. You may look at the Meal Chart to pick different foods that suit your taste buds.

Example Menus

Rest & Recovery Days

160 lbs.

4 Meals Plan

Breakfast: Omelette made w/1 whole Omega-3 egg, 3 egg whites, 3 oz. beef slices, ½ cup sliced red bell pepper, ¼ cup chopped onions; 1 cup green tea

Lunch: 5 oz. grilled chicken breast & ½ cup baked zucchini & 3 cherry tomatoes drizzled with 1 tsp. EVOO on top

Dinner: 7.5 oz. baked tilapia & 12 spears asparagus rolled in 1-1 tsp. coconut oil

Bedtime Snack: Cereal made with ½ cup low-fat cottage cheese, 1 scoop low-carb vanilla protein powder, and 1.5 Tbs. chia seeds; ¾ cup raw broccoli & 3 large baby carrots

5 Meals Plan

Breakfast: Scrambled 1 whole Omega-3 egg, 4 egg whites with ¾ cup raw mushroom and ¼ cup chopped onions; 4 slices turkey bacon; 1 cup green tea

Lunch: 6.75 oz. tuna mixed with ½ Tbs. EVOO mayo on top of Romaine lettuce, ½ cup tomatoes & 1 cup sliced cucumbers

Snack: Protein shake made w/1 scoop low-carb protein powder; 6 large baby carrots; 2 Brazil nut

Dinner: 4 oz. grilled flank steak; ½ cup steamed broccoli drizzled with 1 tsp. flaxseed oil

Bedtime Snack: ⅔ cup Greek yogurt mixed with ⅔ scoop low-carb vanilla protein powder; 3 cherry tomatoes; 1 Tbs. almonds

6 Meals Plan

Breakfast: Omelette w/4 egg whites, 2 turkey bacon, ¼ cup onions & ½ cup sweet bell pepper; ¼ cup avocado slices; 1 c. green tea

Snack: 1 cup tofu fried in ½ tsp. EVOO; ½ cup raw slices of red bell pepper

Lunch: 4 oz. turkey breast chunks served on top of baby spinach & 6 cherry tomatoes drizzled with ½ tsp. flax oil

Snack: 4.5 oz. tuna mixed with ½ Tbs. EVOO mayo & served with ¾ cup raw broccoli flowerets

Dinner: 6 oz. grilled salmon & coleslaw made with ¾ cup shredded cabbage, 1 small carrot stick & 1 Tbs. EVOO mayo

Bedtime Snack: 1 scoop low-carb protein powder (shake), 3 large baby carrots & 7 almonds

Rest & Active Recovery Blueprint

Protein: 21 blocks

Veggies: 4.5 blocks

Fats: 4.5 blocks

REST DAYS – 170 lbs.

The weight loss formula for rest and active recovery days includes healthy proteins, vegetables, and essential fats. We want to eliminate all sugars and starches on rest days as your body will not need them.

4 Meals Menu Plan

Macro	Meal 1	Meal 2	Meal 3	Meal 4	Total
Protein	5	5	6	5	21
Veggie	1	1	1 ½	1	4 ½
Fat	1	1	1	1 ½	4 ½

5 Meals Menu Plan

Macro	Meal 1	Meal 2	Meal 3	Meal 4	Meal 5	Total
Protein	4 ½	4 ½	3	5	4	21
Veggie	1	1	1	1	½	4 ½
Fat	1	½	1	1	1	4 ½

6 Meals Menu Plan

Macro	Meal 1	Meal 2	Meal 3	Meal 4	Meal 5	Meal 6	Total
Protein	3	3	5	3	4	3	21
Veggie	1	½	1	½	1	½	4 ½
Fat	1	½	½	½	1	1	4 ½

Following are example menus for the weight loss formula covering rest and active recovery days for those in the 170 pound category. You may look at the Meal Chart to pick different foods that suit your taste buds.

Example Menus

Rest & Recovery Days

170 lbs.

4 Meals Plan

Breakfast: Omelette made w/1 whole Omega-3 egg, 3 egg whites, 3 oz. beef slices, ½ cup sliced red bell pepper, ¼ cup chopped onions; 1 cup green tea

Lunch: 5 oz. grilled chicken breast & ½ cup baked zucchini & 3 cherry tomatoes drizzled with 1 tsp. EVOO on top

Dinner: 9 oz. baked tilapia & 12 spears asparagus rolled in 1-1 tsp. coconut oil

Bedtime Snack: Cereal made with ½ cup low-fat cottage cheese, 1 scoop low-carb vanilla protein powder, and 1.5 Tbs chia seeds; ¾ cup raw broccoli & 3 large baby carrots

5 Meals Plan

Breakfast: Scrambled 1 whole Omega-3 egg, 4 egg whites with ¾ cup raw mushroom and ¼ cup chopped onions; 4 slices turkey bacon; 1 cup green tea

Lunch: 6.75 oz. tuna mixed with ½ Tbs. EVOO mayo on top of Romaine lettuce & ½ cup tomatoes, 1 cup sliced cucumbers

Snack: Protein shake made w/1 scoop low-carb protein powder; 6 large baby carrots; 2 Brazil nut

Dinner: 5 oz. grilled flank steak; ½ cup steamed broccoli drizzled with 1 tsp. flaxseed oil

Bedtime Snack: ⅔ cup Greek yogurt mixed with ⅔ scoop low-carb vanilla protein powder; 3 cherry tomatoes; 1 Tbs. almonds

6 Meals Plan

Breakfast: Omelette w/4 egg whites, 2 turkey bacon, ¼ cup onions & ½ cup sweet bell pepper; ¼ cup avocado slices; 1 c. green tea

Snack: 1 cup tofu fried in ½ tsp. EVOO; ½ cup raw slices of red bell pepper

Lunch: 5 oz. turkey breast chunks served on top of baby spinach & 6 cherry tomatoes drizzled with ½ tsp. flax oil

Snack: 4.5 oz. tuna mixed with ½ Tbs. EVOO mayo & served with ¾ cup raw broccoli flowerets

Dinner: 6 oz. grilled salmon & coleslaw made with ¾ cup shredded cabbage, 1 small carrot stick & 1 Tbs. EVOO mayo

Bedtime Snack: 1 scoop low-carb protein powder (shake), 3 large baby carrots & 7 almonds

<table>
<tr><td colspan="2">

Rest & Active Recovery Blueprint

Protein: 22.5 blocks

Veggies: 5 blocks

Fats: 5 blocks

</td></tr>
</table>

REST DAYS – 180 lbs.

The weight loss formula for rest and active recovery days includes healthy proteins, vegetables, and essential fats. We want to eliminate all sugars and starches on rest days as your body will not need them.

4 Meals Menu Plan

Macro	Meal 1	Meal 2	Meal 3	Meal 4	Total
Protein	5 ½	6	6	5	22 ½
Veggie	1	1	2	1	5
Fat	1	1	1 ½	1 ½	5

5 Meals Menu Plan

Macro	Meal 1	Meal 2	Meal 3	Meal 4	Meal 5	Total
Protein	4 ½	4 ½	4	5 ½	4	22 ½
Veggie	1	1	1	1	1	5
Fat	1	1	1	1	1	5

6 Meals Menu Plan

Macro	Meal 1	Meal 2	Meal 3	Meal 4	Meal 5	Meal 6	Total
Protein	3	3	5	4	4	3 ½	22 ½
Veggie	1	½	1	½	1	1	5
Fat	1	½	1	½	1	1	5

Following are example menus for the weight loss formula covering rest and active recovery days for those in the 180 pound category. You may look at the Meal Chart to pick different foods that suit your taste buds.

Example Menus

Rest & Recovery Days

180 lbs.

4 Meals Plan

Breakfast: Omelette made w/1 whole Omega-3 egg, 3 egg whites, 3.5 oz. beef slices, ½ cup sliced red bell pepper, ¼ cup chopped onions; 1 cup green tea

Lunch: 6 oz. grilled chicken breast & ½ cup baked zucchini & 3 cherry tomatoes drizzled with 1 tsp. EVOO on top

Dinner: 9 oz. baked tilapia & 16 spears asparagus rolled in 1-1½ tsp. coconut oil

Bedtime Snack: Cereal made with ½ cup low-fat cottage cheese, 1 scoop low-carb vanilla protein powder, and 1.5 Tbs chia seeds; ¾ cup raw broccoli & 6 large baby carrots

5 Meals Plan

Breakfast: Scrambled 1 whole Omega-3 egg, 4 egg whites with ¾ cup raw mushroom and ¼ cup chopped onions; 4 slices turkey bacon; 1 cup green tea

Lunch: 6.75 oz. tuna mixed with 1 Tbs. EVOO mayo on top of Romaine lettuce, ½ cup tomatoes & 1 cup sliced cucumbers

Snack: Protein shake with 1-⅓ scoop low-carb protein powder; 6 large baby carrots; 2 Brazil nut

Dinner: 5.5 oz. grilled flank steak; ½ cup steamed broccoli drizzled with 1 tsp. flaxseed oil

Bedtime Snack: ⅔ cup Greek yogurt mixed with ⅔ scoop low-carb vanilla protein powder; 6 cherry tomatoes; 1 Tbs. almonds

6 Meals Plan

Breakfast: Omelette w/4 egg whites, 2 turkey bacon, ¼ cup onions & ½ cup sweet bell pepper; ¼ cup avocado slices; 1 c. green tea

Snack: 1 cup tofu fried in ½ tsp. EVOO; ½ cup raw slices of red bell pepper

Lunch: 5 oz. turkey breast chunks served on top of baby spinach & 1 cup cucumbers, drizzled with 1 tsp. flax oil

Snack: 6 oz. tuna mixed with ½ Tbs. EVOO mayo & served with ¾ cup raw broccoli floweret

Dinner: 6 oz. grilled salmon & coleslaw made with ¾ cup shredded cabbage, 1 small carrot stick & 1 Tbs. EVOO mayo

Bedtime Snack: 1 heaping scoop low-carb protein powder (shake), 6 large baby carrots & 7 almonds

REST DAYS – 190 lbs.

The weight loss formula for rest and active recovery days includes healthy proteins, vegetables, and essential fats. We want to eliminate all sugars and starches on rest days as your body will not need them.

4 Meals Menu Plan

Macro	Meal 1	Meal 2	Meal 3	Meal 4	Total
Protein	6	6	6	6	24
Veggie	1	1	2	1	5
Fat	1	1	1 ½	1 ½	5

5 Meals Menu Plan

Macro	Meal 1	Meal 2	Meal 3	Meal 4	Meal 5	Total
Protein	5	5	4	6	4	24
Veggie	1	1	1	1	1	5
Fat	1	1	1	1	1	5

6 Meals Menu Plan

Macro	Meal 1	Meal 2	Meal 3	Meal 4	Meal 5	Meal 6	Total
Protein	4	3	5	4	4	4	24
Veggie	1	½	1	½	1	1	5
Fat	1	½	1	½	1	1	5

Following are example menus for the weight loss formula covering rest and active recovery days for those in the 190 pound category. You may look at the Meal Chart to pick different foods that suit your taste buds.

Example Menus

Rest & Recovery Days

190 lbs.

4 Meals Plan

Breakfast: Omelette made w/1 whole Omega-3 egg, 3 egg whites, 4 oz. beef slices, ½ cup sliced red bell pepper, ¼ cup chopped onions; 1 cup green tea

Lunch: 6 oz. grilled chicken breast & ½ cup baked zucchini & 3 cherry tomatoes drizzled with 1 tsp. EVOO on top

Dinner: 9 oz. baked tilapia & 16 spears asparagus rolled in 1-1½ tsp. coconut oil

Bedtime Snack: Cereal made with ¾ cup low-fat cottage cheese, 1 scoop low-carb vanilla protein powder, and 1.5 Tbs. chia seeds; ¾ cup raw broccoli & 3 large baby carrots

5 Meals Plan

Breakfast: Scrambled 1 whole Omega-3 egg, 5 egg whites with ¾ cup raw mushroom and ¼ cup chopped onions; 4 slices turkey bacon; 1 cup green tea

Lunch: 7.5 oz. tuna mixed with 1 Tbs. EVOO mayo on top of Romaine lettuce, ½ cup tomatoes & 1 cup sliced cucumbers

Snack: Protein shake made with 1-⅓ scoop low-carb protein powder; 6 large baby carrots; 2 Brazil nut

Dinner: 6 oz. grilled flank steak; ½ cup steamed broccoli drizzled with 1 tsp. flaxseed oil

Bedtime Snack: ⅔ cup Greek yogurt mixed with ⅔ scoop low-carb vanilla protein powder; 6 cherry tomatoes; 1 Tbs. almonds

6 Meals Plan

Breakfast: Omelette w/4 egg whites, 4 turkey bacon, ¼ cup onions & ½ cup sweet bell pepper; ¼ cup avocado slices; 1 c. green tea

Snack: 1 cup tofu fried in ½ tsp. EVOO; ½ cup raw slices of red bell pepper

Lunch: 5 oz. turkey breast chunks served on top of baby spinach & 6 cherry tomatoes, drizzled with 1 tsp. flax oil

Snack: 6 oz. tuna mixed with ½ Tbs. EVOO mayo & served with ¾ cup raw broccoli flowerets

Dinner: 6 oz. grilled salmon & coleslaw made with ¾ cup shredded cabbage, 1 small carrot stick & 1 Tbs. EVOO mayo

Bedtime Snack: 1-⅓ scoops low-carb protein powder (shake), 6 large baby carrots & 7 almonds

| **Rest & Active Recovery Blueprint**

Protein: 25 blocks

Veggies: 5.5 blocks

Fats: 5.5 blocks |

REST DAYS – 200 lbs.

The weight loss formula for rest and active recovery days includes healthy proteins, vegetables, and essential fats. We want to eliminate all sugars and starches on rest days as your body will not need them.

4 Meals Menu Plan

Macro	Meal 1	Meal 2	Meal 3	Meal 4	Total
Protein	6	6	7	6	25
Veggie	1 ½	1	2	1	5 ½
Fat	1 ½	1	1 ½	1 ½	5 ½

5 Meals Menu Plan

Macro	Meal 1	Meal 2	Meal 3	Meal 4	Meal 5	Total
Protein	4 ½	4 ½	6	6	4	25
Veggie	1	1	1	1 ½	1	5 ½
Fat	1	1	1	1	1 ½	5 ½

6 Meals Menu Plan

Macro	Meal 1	Meal 2	Meal 3	Meal 4	Meal 5	Meal 6	Total
Protein	4	3	5	4	5	4	25
Veggie	1	½	1	1	1	1	5 ½
Fat	1	½	1	1	1	1	5 ½

Following are example menus for the weight loss formula covering rest and active recovery days for those in the 200 pound category. You may look at the Meal Chart to pick different foods that suit your taste buds.

4 Meals Plan

Breakfast: Omelette made w/1 whole Omega-3 egg, 3 egg whites, 4 oz. beef slices, ½ cup sliced red bell pepper, ¼ cup chopped onions & ½ cup chopped tomatoes - cooked in ½ tsp. EVOO; 1 cup green tea

Lunch: 6 oz. grilled chicken breast & ½ cup baked zucchini & 3 cherry tomatoes drizzled with 1 tsp. EVOO on top

Dinner: 10.5 oz. baked tilapia & 16 spears asparagus rolled in 1-½ tsp. coconut oil

Bedtime Snack: Cereal made with ¾ cup low-fat cottage cheese, 1 scoop low-carb vanilla protein powder, and 1.5 Tbs. chia seeds; ¾ cup raw broccoli & 3 large baby carrots

5 Meals Plan

Breakfast: Scrambled 1 whole Omega-3 egg, 4 egg whites with ¾ cup raw mushroom and ¼ cup chopped onions; 4 slices turkey bacon; 1 cup green tea

Lunch: 6.75 oz. tuna mixed with 1 Tbs. EVOO mayo on top of Romaine lettuce, ½ cup tomatoes & 1 cup sliced cucumbers

Snack: Protein shake made with 2 scoops slow-carb protein powder; 6 large baby carrots; 2 Brazil nut

Dinner: 6 oz. grilled flank steak; ¾ cup steamed broccoli drizzled with 1 tsp. flaxseed oil

Bedtime Snack: ⅔ cup Greek yogurt mixed with ⅔ scoop low-carb vanilla protein powder; 6 cherry tomatoes; 1-½ Tbs. almonds

6 Meals Plan

Breakfast: Omelette w/4 egg whites, 4 turkey bacon, ¼ cup onions & ½ cup sweet bell pepper; ¼ cup avocado slices; 1 c. green tea

Snack: 1 cup tofu fried in ½ tsp. EVOO; ½ cup raw slices of red bell pepper

Lunch: 5 oz. turkey breast chunks served on top of baby spinach 6 cherry tomatoes, drizzled with 1 tsp. flax oil

Snack: 6 oz. tuna mixed with 1 Tbs. EVOO mayo & served with ¾ cup raw broccoli flowerets & 3 baby carrots

Dinner: 7.5 oz. grilled salmon & coleslaw made with ¾ cup shredded cabbage, 1 small carrot stick & 1 Tbs. EVOO mayo

Bedtime Snack: 1-⅓ scoops low-carb protein powder (shake), 6 large baby carrots & 7 almonds

Rest & Active Recovery Blueprint

Protein: 26 blocks

Veggies: 5.5 blocks

Fats: 5.5 blocks

REST DAYS – 210 lbs.

The weight loss formula for rest and active recovery days includes healthy proteins, vegetables, and essential fats. We want to eliminate all sugars and starches on rest days as your body will not need them.

4 Meals Menu Plan

Macro	Meal 1	Meal 2	Meal 3	Meal 4	Total
Protein	6	6	7	7	26
Veggie	1 ½	1	2	1	5 ½
Fat	1 ½	1	1 ½	1 ½	5 ½

5 Meals Menu Plan

Macro	Meal 1	Meal 2	Meal 3	Meal 4	Meal 5	Total
Protein	4 ½	4 ½	6	6	5	26
Veggie	1	1	1	1 ½	1	5 ½
Fat	1	1	1	1	1 ½	5 ½

6 Meals Menu Plan

Macro	Meal 1	Meal 2	Meal 3	Meal 4	Meal 5	Meal 6	Total
Protein	4	4	5	4	5	4	26
Veggie	1	½	1	1	1	1	5 ½
Fat	1	½	1	1	1	1	5 ½

Following are example menus for the weight loss formula covering rest and active recovery days for those in the 210 pound category. You may look at the Meal Chart to pick different foods that suit your taste buds.

Example Menus

Rest & Recovery Days

210 lbs.

4 Meals Plan

Breakfast: Omelette made w/1 whole Omega-3 egg, 3 egg whites, 4 oz. beef slices, ½ cup sliced red bell pepper, ¼ cup chopped onions & ½ cup chopped tomatoes - cooked in ½ tsp. EVOO; 1 cup green tea

Lunch: 6 oz. grilled chicken breast & ½ cup baked zucchini & 3 cherry tomatoes drizzled with 1 tsp. EVOO on top

Dinner: 10.5 oz. baked tilapia & 16 spears asparagus rolled in 1-½ tsp. coconut oil

Bedtime Snack: Cereal made with 1 cup low-fat cottage cheese, 1 scoop low-carb vanilla protein powder, and 1.5 Tbs. chia seeds; ¾ cup raw broccoli & 3 large baby carrots

5 Meals Plan

Breakfast: Scrambled 1 whole Omega-3 egg, 4 egg whites with ¾ cup raw mushroom and ¼ cup chopped onions; 4 slices turkey bacon; 1 cup green tea

Lunch: 6.75 oz. tuna mixed with 1 Tbs. EVOO mayo on top of Romaine lettuce, ½ cup tomatoes & 1 cup sliced cucumbers

Snack: Protein shake made with 2 scoops low-carb protein powder; 6 large baby carrots; 2 Brazil nut

Dinner: 6 oz. grilled flank steak; ¾ cup steamed broccoli drizzled with 1 tsp. flaxseed oil

Bedtime Snack: ⅔ cup Greek yogurt mixed with 1 scoop low-carb vanilla protein powder; 6 cherry tomatoes; 1-½ Tbs. almonds

6 Meals Plan

Breakfast: Omelette w/4 egg whites, 4 turkey bacon, ¼ cup onions & ½ cup sweet bell pepper; ¼ cup avocado slices; 1 c. green tea

Snack: 1-⅓ cup tofu fried in ½ tsp. EVOO; ½ cup raw slices of red bell pepper

Lunch: 5 oz. turkey breast chunks served on top of baby spinach & 6 cherry tomatoes drizzled with 1 tsp. flax oil

Snack: 6 oz. tuna mixed with 1 Tbs. EVOO mayo & served with ¾ cup raw broccoli flowerets & 3 baby carrots

Dinner: 7.5 oz. grilled salmon & coleslaw made with ¾ cup shredded cabbage, 1 small carrot stick & 1 Tbs. EVOO mayo

Bedtime Snack: 1-⅓ scoops low-carb protein powder (shake), 6 large baby carrots & 7 almonds

Rest & Active Recovery Blueprint
Protein: 27.5 blocks
Veggies: 6 blocks
Fats: 6 blocks

The weight loss formula for rest and active recovery days includes healthy proteins, vegetables, and essential fats. We want to eliminate all sugars and starches on rest days as your body will not need them.

4 Meals Menu Plan

Macro	Meal 1	Meal 2	Meal 3	Meal 4	Total
Protein	7	6	7	7	27
Veggie	1 ½	1 ½	2	1	6
Fat	1 ½	1 ½	1 ½	1 ½	6

5 Meals Menu Plan

Macro	Meal 1	Meal 2	Meal 3	Meal 4	Meal 5	Total
Protein	5	5	6	6	5	27
Veggie	1 ½	1	1	1 ½	1	6
Fat	1	1	1	1 ½	1 ½	6

6 Meals Menu Plan

Macro	Meal 1	Meal 2	Meal 3	Meal 4	Meal 5	Meal 6	Total
Protein	4	4	5	4	6	4	27
Veggie	1	1	1	1	1	1	6
Fat	1	1	1	1	1	1	6

Following are example menus for the weight loss formula covering rest and active recovery days for those in the 220 pound category. You may look at the Meal Chart to pick different foods that suit your taste buds.

Example Menus

Rest & Recovery Days

220 lbs.

4 Meals Plan

Breakfast: Omelette made w/1 whole Omega-3 egg, 5 egg whites, 4 oz. beef slices, ½ cup sliced red bell pepper, ¼ cup chopped onions & ½ cup chopped tomatoes - cooked in ½ tsp. EVOO; 1 cup green tea

Lunch: 6 oz. grilled chicken breast & ½ cup baked zucchini & 6 cherry tomatoes with 1-½ tsp. EVOO drizzled on top

Dinner: 10.5 oz. baked tilapia & 16 spears asparagus rolled in 1-½ tsp. coconut oil

Bedtime Snack: Cereal made with 1 cup low-fat cottage cheese, 1 scoop low-carb vanilla protein powder, and 1.5 Tbs. chia seeds; ¾ cup raw broccoli; 3 large baby carrots

5 Meals Plan

Breakfast: Scrambled 1 whole Omega-3 egg, 5 egg whites with ¾ cup raw mushroom , ½ cup chopped tomatoes, and ¼ cup chopped onions; 4 slices turkey bacon; 1 cup green tea

Lunch: 7.5 oz. tuna mixed with 1 Tbs. EVOO mayo on top of Romaine lettuce, ½ cup tomatoes & 1 cup sliced cucumbers

Snack: Protein shake made with 2 scoops low-carb protein powder; 6 large baby carrots; 2 Brazil nut

Dinner: 6 oz. grilled flank steak; ¾ cup steamed broccoli drizzled with 1-½ tsp. flaxseed oil

Bedtime Snack: ⅔ cup Greek yogurt mixed with 1 scoop low-carb vanilla protein powder; 6 cherry tomatoes; 1-½ Tbs. almonds

6 Meals Plan

Breakfast: Omelette w/4 egg whites, 4 turkey bacon, ¼ cup onions & ½ cup sweet bell pepper; ¼ cup avocado slices; 1 c. green tea

Snack: 1-⅓ cup tofu fried in 1 tsp. EVOO; 1 cup raw slices of red bell pepper

Lunch: 5 oz. turkey breast chunks served on top of baby spinach & 6 cherry tomatoes drizzled with 1 tsp. flax oil

Snack: 6 oz. tuna mixed with 1 Tbs. EVOO mayo & served with ¾ cup raw broccoli flowerets & 3 baby carrots

Dinner: 9 oz. grilled salmon & coleslaw made with ¾ cup shredded cabbage, 1 small carrot stick & 1 Tbs. EVOO mayo

Bedtime Snack: 1-⅓ scoops low-carb protein powder (shake), 6 large baby carrots & 7 almonds

Rest & Active Recovery Blueprint

Protein: 29 blocks

Veggies: 6 blocks

Fats: 6 blocks

REST DAYS – 230 lbs.

The weight loss formula for rest and active recovery days includes healthy proteins, vegetables, and essential fats. We want to eliminate all sugars and starches on rest days as your body will not need them.

4 Meals Menu Plan

Macro	Meal 1	Meal 2	Meal 3	Meal 4	Total
Protein	7	7	8	7	29
Veggie	1 ½	1 ½	2	1	6
Fat	1 ½	1 ½	1 ½	1 ½	6

5 Meals Menu Plan

Macro	Meal 1	Meal 2	Meal 3	Meal 4	Meal 5	Total
Protein	5	5	6	7	6	29
Veggie	1 ½	1	1	1 ½	1	6
Fat	1	1	1	1 ½	1 ½	6

6 Meals Menu Plan

Macro	Meal 1	Meal 2	Meal 3	Meal 4	Meal 5	Meal 6	Total
Protein	4	4	5	5	6	5	29
Veggie	1	1	1	1	1	1	6
Fat	1	1	1	1	1	1	6

Following are example menus for the weight loss formula covering rest and active recovery days for those in the 230 pound category. You may look at the Meal Chart to pick different foods that suit your taste buds.

Example Menus

Rest & Recovery Days

230 lbs.

4 Meals Plan

Breakfast: Omelette made w/1 whole Omega-3 egg, 5 egg whites, 4 oz. beef slices, ½ cup sliced red bell pepper, ¼ cup chopped onions & ½ cup chopped tomatoes - cooked in ½ tsp. EVOO; 1 cup green tea

Lunch: 7 oz. grilled chicken breast & ½ cup baked zucchini & 6 cherry tomatoes with 1-½ tsp. EVOO drizzled on top

Dinner: 12 oz. baked tilapia & 16 spears asparagus rolled in 1-½ tsp. coconut oil

Bedtime Snack: Cereal made with 1 cup low-fat cottage cheese, 1 scoop low-carb vanilla protein powder, and 1.5 Tbs. chia seeds; ¾ cup raw broccoli & 3 large baby carrots

5 Meals Plan

Breakfast: Scrambled 1 whole Omega-3 egg, 5 egg whites with ¾ cup raw mushroom , ½ cup chopped tomatoes, and ¼ cup chopped onions; 4 slices turkey bacon; 1 cup green tea

Lunch: 7.5 oz. tuna mixed with 1 Tbs. EVOO mayo on top of Romaine lettuce, ½ cup tomatoes & 1 cup sliced cucumbers

Snack: Protein shake made with 2 scoops low-carb protein powder; 6 large baby carrots; 2 Brazil nut

Dinner: 7 oz. grilled flank steak; ¾ cup steamed broccoli drizzled with 1-½ tsp. flaxseed oil

Bedtime Snack: 1 cup Greek yogurt mixed with 1 scoop low-carb vanilla protein powder; 6 cherry tomatoes; 1-½ Tbs. almonds

6 Meals Plan

Breakfast: Omelette w/4 egg whites, 4 turkey bacon, ¼ cup onions & ½ cup sweet bell pepper; ¼ cup avocado slices; 1 c. green tea

Snack: 1-⅓ cup tofu fried in 1 tsp. EVOO; 1 cup raw slices of red bell pepper

Lunch: 5 oz. turkey breast chunks served on top of baby spinach & 6 cherry tomatoes, drizzled with 1 tsp. flax oil

Snack: 7.5 oz. tuna mixed with 1 Tbs. EVOO mayo & served with ¾ cup raw broccoli flowerets & 3 baby carrots

Dinner: 9 oz. grilled salmon & coleslaw made with ¾ cup shredded cabbage, 1 small carrot stick & 1 Tbs. EVOO mayo

Bedtime Snack: 1-⅔ scoops low-carb protein powder (shake), 6 large baby carrots & 7 almonds

Rest & Active Recovery Blueprint

Protein: 30 blocks

Veggies: 6.5 blocks

Fats: 6.5 blocks

The weight loss formula for rest and active recovery days includes healthy proteins, vegetables, and essential fats. We want to eliminate all sugars and starches on rest days as your body will not need them.

4 Meals Menu Plan

Macro	Meal 1	Meal 2	Meal 3	Meal 4	Total
Protein	7	8	8	7	30
Veggie	1 ½	1 ½	2	1 ½	6 ½
Fat	1 ½	1 ½	1 ½	2	6 ½

5 Meals Menu Plan

Macro	Meal 1	Meal 2	Meal 3	Meal 4	Meal 5	Total
Protein	5	6	6	7	6	30
Veggie	1 ½	1	1	2	1	6 ½
Fat	1	1	1	1 ½	2	6 ½

6 Meals Menu Plan

Macro	Meal 1	Meal 2	Meal 3	Meal 4	Meal 5	Meal 6	Total
Protein	4	4	5	5	7	5	30
Veggie	1	1	1	1	1 ½	1	6 ½
Fat	1	1	1	1	1	1 ½	6 ½

Following are example menus for the weight loss formula covering rest and active recovery days for those in the 240 pound category. You may look at the Meal Chart to pick different foods that suit your taste buds.

Example Menus

Rest & Recovery Days

240 lbs.

4 Meals Plan

Breakfast: Omelette made w/1 whole Omega-3 egg, 5 egg whites, 4 oz. beef slices, ½ cup sliced red bell pepper, ¼ cup chopped onions & ½ cup chopped tomatoes - cooked in ½ tsp. EVOO; 1 cup green tea

Lunch: 8 oz. grilled chicken breast & ½ cup baked zucchini & 6 cherry tomatoes drizzled with 1-½ tsp. EVOO on top

Dinner: 12 oz. baked tilapia & 16 spears asparagus rolled in 1-½ tsp. coconut oil

Bedtime Snack: Cereal made with 1 cup low-fat cottage cheese, 1 scoop low-carb vanilla protein powder, and 2 Tbs. chia seeds; ¾ cup raw broccoli & 6 large baby carrots

5 Meals Plan

Breakfast: Scrambled 1 whole Omega-3 egg, 5 egg whites with ¾ cup raw mushroom , ½ cup chopped tomatoes, and ¼ cup chopped onions; 4 slices turkey bacon; 1 cup green tea

Lunch: 9 oz. tuna mixed with 1 Tbs. EVOO mayo on top of Romaine lettuce, ½ cup tomatoes & 1 cup sliced cucumbers

Snack: Protein shake made with 2 scoops low-carb protein powder; 6 large baby carrots; 2 Brazil nut

Dinner: 7 oz. grilled flank steak; 1 cup steamed broccoli drizzled with 1.5 tsp. flaxseed oil

Bedtime Snack: 1 cup Greek yogurt mixed with 1 scoop low-carb vanilla protein powder; 6 cherry tomatoes; 2 Tbs. almonds

6 Meals Plan

Breakfast: Omelette w/4 egg whites, 4 turkey bacon, ¼ cup onions & ½ cup sweet bell pepper; ¼ cup avocado slices; 1 c. green tea

Snack: 1-⅓ cup tofu fried in 1 tsp. EVOO; 1 cup raw slices of red bell pepper

Lunch: 5 oz. turkey breast chunks served on top of baby spinach & 6 cherry tomatoes drizzled with 1 tsp. flax oil

Snack: 7.5 oz. tuna mixed with 1 Tbs. EVOO mayo & served with ¾ cup raw broccoli flowerets & 3 baby carrots

Dinner: 10.5 oz. salmon & coleslaw made with ¾ cup shredded cabbage, 1 small carrot stick & 1 Tbs. EVOO mayo

Bedtime Snack: 1-⅔ scoops low-carb protein powder (shake), 6 large baby carrots & 11 almonds

Rest & Active Recovery Blueprint
Protein: 31 blocks
Veggies: 6.5 blocks
Fats: 6.5 blocks

REST DAYS – 250 lbs.

The weight loss formula for rest and active recovery days includes healthy proteins, vegetables, and essential fats. We want to eliminate all sugars and starches on rest days as your body will not need them.

4 Meals Menu Plan

Macro	Meal 1	Meal 2	Meal 3	Meal 4	Total
Protein	7	8	8	8	31
Veggie	1 ½	1 ½	2	1 ½	6 ½
Fat	1 ½	1 ½	1 ½	2	6 ½

5 Meals Menu Plan

Macro	Meal 1	Meal 2	Meal 3	Meal 4	Meal 5	Total
Protein	5	6	6	8	6	31
Veggie	1 ½	1	1	2	1	6 ½
Fat	1	1	1	1 ½	2	6 ½

6 Meals Menu Plan

Macro	Meal 1	Meal 2	Meal 3	Meal 4	Meal 5	Meal 6	Total
Protein	4	4	6	5	7	5	31
Veggie	1	1	1	1	1 ½	1	6 ½
Fat	1	1	1	1	1	1 ½	6 ½

Following are example menus for the weight loss formula covering rest and active recovery days for those in the 250 pound category. You may look at the Meal Chart to pick different foods that suit your taste buds.

Example Menus

Rest & Recovery Days

250 lbs.

4 Meals Plan

Breakfast: Omelette made w/1 whole Omega-3 egg, 5 egg whites, 4 oz. beef slices, ½ cup sliced red bell pepper, ¼ cup chopped onions & ½ cup chopped tomatoes - cooked in ½ tsp. EVOO; 1 cup green tea

Lunch: 8 oz. grilled chicken breast & ½ cup baked zucchini & 6 cherry tomatoes drizzled with 1-½ tsp. EVOO on top

Dinner: 12 oz. baked tilapia & 16 spears asparagus rolled in 1-½ tsp. coconut oil

Bedtime Snack: Cereal made with 1 cup low-fat cottage cheese, 1-⅓ scoops low-carb vanilla protein powder, and 2 TBS. chia seeds; ¾ cup raw broccoli & 6 large baby carrots

5 Meals Plan

Breakfast: Scrambled 1 whole Omega-3 egg, 5 egg whites with ¾ cup raw mushroom, ½ cup cherry tomatoes, and ¼ cup chopped onions; 4 slices turkey bacon; 1 cup green tea

Lunch: 9 oz. tuna mixed with 1 Tbs. EVOO mayo on top of Romaine lettuce, ½ cup tomatoes & 1 cup sliced cucumbers

Snack: Protein shake made with 2 scoops low-carb protein powder; 6 large baby carrots; 2 Brazil nut

Dinner: 8 oz. grilled flank steak; 1 cup steamed broccoli drizzled with 1-½ tsp. flaxseed oil

Bedtime Snack: 1 cup Greek yogurt mixed with 1 scoop low-carb vanilla protein powder; 6 cherry tomatoes; 2 Tbs. almonds

6 Meals Plan

Breakfast: Omelette w/4 egg whites, 4 turkey bacon, ¼ cup onions & ½ cup sweet bell pepper; ¼ cup avocado slices; 1 c. green tea

Snack: 1-⅓ cup tofu fried in 1 tsp. EVOO; 1 cup raw slices of red bell pepper

Lunch: 6 oz. turkey breast chunks served on top of baby spinach & 6 cherry tomatoes drizzled with 1 tsp. flax oil

Snack: 7.5 oz. tuna mixed with 1 Tbs. EVOO mayo & served with ¾ cup raw broccoli flowerets & 3 baby carrots

Dinner: 10.5 oz. salmon & coleslaw made with ¾ cup shredded cabbage, 1 small carrot stick & 1.5 Tbs. EVOO mayo

Bedtime Snack: 1-⅔ scoops low-carb protein powder (shake), 6 large baby carrots & 11 almonds

Rest & Active Recovery Blueprint

Protein: 32.5 blocks

Veggies: 7 blocks

Fats: 7 blocks

The weight loss formula for rest and active recovery days includes healthy proteins, vegetables, and essential fats. We want to eliminate all sugars and starches on rest days as your body will not need them.

4 Meals Menu Plan

Macro	Meal 1	Meal 2	Meal 3	Meal 4	Total
Protein	8	8 ½	8	8	32 ½
Veggie	2	1 ½	2	1 ½	7
Fat	2	1 ½	1 ½	2	7

5 Meals Menu Plan

Macro	Meal 1	Meal 2	Meal 3	Meal 4	Meal 5	Total
Protein	5	6	7	8 ½	6	32 ½
Veggie	2	1	1	2	1	7
Fat	1	1	1	2	2	7

6 Meals Menu Plan

Macro	Meal 1	Meal 2	Meal 3	Meal 4	Meal 5	Meal 6	Total
Protein	4	4 ½	7	5	7	5	32 ½
Veggie	1	1	1	1	2	1	7
Fat	1	1	1	1	1	2	7

Following are example menus for the weight loss formula covering rest and active recovery days for those in the 260 pound category. You may look at the Meal Chart to pick different foods that suit your taste buds.

Example Menus

Rest & Recovery Days

260 lbs.

4 Meals Plan

Breakfast: Omelette made w/1 whole Omega-3 egg, 5 egg whites, 5 oz. beef slices, 1 cup sliced red bell pepper, ¼ cup chopped onions & ½ cup chopped tomatoes - cooked in 2 tsp. EVOO; 1 cup green tea

Lunch: 8 .5 oz. grilled chicken breast & ½ cup baked zucchini & 6 cherry tomatoes drizzled with 1-½ tsp. EVOO on top

Dinner: 12 oz. baked tilapia & 16 spears asparagus rolled in 1-½ tsp. coconut oil

Bedtime Snack: Cereal made with 1 cup low-fat cottage cheese, 1-⅓ scoops low-carb vanilla protein powder, and 2 Tbs. chia seeds; ¾ cup raw broccoli & 6 large baby carrots

5 Meals Plan

Breakfast: Scrambled 1 whole Omega-3 egg, 5 egg whites with ¾ cup raw mushroom, ½ cup chopped tomatoes & ¼ cup chopped onions; 4 slices turkey bacon; ½ cup low-sodium V-8; 1 cup green tea

Lunch: 9 oz. tuna mixed with 1 Tbs. EVOO mayo on top of Romaine lettuce, ½ cup tomatoes & 1 cup sliced cucumbers

Snack: Protein shake made with 2-⅓ scoops low-carb protein powder; 6 large baby carrots; 2 Brazil nut

Dinner: 8.5 oz. grilled flank steak; 1 cup steamed broccoli drizzled with 2 tsp. flaxseed oil

Bedtime Snack: 1 cup Greek yogurt mixed with 1 scoop low-carb vanilla protein powder; 6 cherry tomatoes; 2 Tbs. almonds

6 Meals Plan

Breakfast: Omelette w/4 egg whites, 4 turkey bacon, ¼ cup onions & ½ cup sweet bell pepper; ¼ cup avocado slices; 1 c. green tea

Snack: 1-½ cups tofu fried in 1 tsp. EVOO; 1 cup raw slices of beil pepper

Lunch: 7 oz. turkey breast chunks served on top of baby spinach & 6 cherry tomatoes drizzled with 1 tsp. flax oil

Snack: 7.5 oz. tuna mixed with 1 Tbs. EVOO mayo & served with ¾ cup raw broccoli flowerets & 3 baby carrots

Dinner: 10.5 oz. salmon & coleslaw made with ¾ cup shredded cabbage, 2 small carrot stick & 1 Tbs. EVOO mayo

Bedtime Snack: 1-⅔ scoops low-carb protein powder (shake), 6 large baby carrots & 14 almonds

Rest & Active Recovery Blueprint
Protein: 34 blocks
Veggies: 7 blocks
Fats: 7 blocks

The weight loss formula for rest and active recovery days includes healthy proteins, vegetables, and essential fats. We want to eliminate all sugars and starches on rest days as your body will not need them.

4 Meals Menu Plan

Macro	Meal 1	Meal 2	Meal 3	Meal 4	Total
Protein	8	9	8	9	34
Veggie	2	1 ½	2	1 ½	7
Fat	2	1 ½	1 ½	2	7

5 Meals Menu Plan

Macro	Meal 1	Meal 2	Meal 3	Meal 4	Meal 5	Total
Protein	5	6	7	8 ½	7 ½	34
Veggie	2	1	1	2	1	7
Fat	1	1	1	2	2	7

6 Meals Menu Plan

Macro	Meal 1	Meal 2	Meal 3	Meal 4	Meal 5	Meal 6	Total
Protein	4	4 ½	8	5	7	5 ½	34
Veggie	1	1	1	1	2	1	7
Fat	1	1	1	1	1	2	7

Following are example menus for the weight loss formula covering rest and active recovery days for those in the 270 pound category. You may look at the Meal Chart to pick different foods that suit your taste buds.

Example Menus

Rest & Recovery Days

270 lbs.

4 Meals Plan

Breakfast: Omelette made w/1 whole Omega-3 egg, 5 egg whites, 5 oz. beef slices, 1 cup sliced red bell pepper, ¼ cup chopped onions & ½ cup chopped tomatoes - cooked in 2 tsp. EVOO; 1 cup green tea

Lunch: 9 oz. grilled chicken breast & ½ cup baked zucchini & 6 cherry tomatoes drizzled with 1-½ tsp. EVOO on top

Dinner: 12 oz. baked tilapia & 16 spears asparagus rolled in 1-½ tsp. coconut oil

Bedtime Snack: Cereal made with 1 cup low-fat cottage cheese, 1-⅔ scoops low-carb vanilla protein powder, and 2 Tbs. chia seeds; ¾ cup raw broccoli & 6 large baby carrots

5 Meals Plan

Breakfast: Scrambled 1 whole Omega-3 egg, 5 egg whites with ¾ cup raw mushroom , ½ cup chopped tomatoes & ¼ cup chopped onions; 4 slices turkey bacon; ½ cup low-sodium V-8; 1 cup green tea

Lunch: 9 oz. tuna mixed with 1 Tbs. EVOO mayo on top of Romaine lettuce, ½ cup tomatoes & 1 cup sliced cucumbers

Snack: Protein shake made with 2-⅓ scoops low-carb protein powder; 6 large baby carrots; 2 Brazil nut

Dinner: 8.5 oz. grilled flank steak; 1 cup steamed broccoli drizzled with 2 tsp. flaxseed oil

Bedtime Snack: 1 cup Greek yogurt mixed with 1.5 scoops low-carb vanilla protein powder; 6 cherry tomatoes; 2 Tbs. almonds

6 Meals Plan

Breakfast: Omelette w/4 egg whites, 4 turkey bacon, ¼ cup onions & ½ cup sweet bell pepper; ¼ cup avocado slices; 1 c. green tea

Snack: 1-½ cups tofu fried in 1 tsp. EVOO; 1 cup raw slices of bell pepper

Lunch: 8 oz. turkey breast chunks served on top of baby spinach & 6 cherry tomatoes drizzled with 1 tsp. flax oil

Snack: 7.5 oz. tuna mixed with 1 Tbs. EVOO mayo & served with ¾ cup raw broccoli flowerets & 3 baby carrots

Dinner: 10.5 oz. salmon & coleslaw made with ¾ cup shredded cabbage, 2 small carrot stick & 1 Tbs. EVOO mayo

Bedtime Snack: 1-¾ scoops low-carb protein powder (shake), 6 large baby carrots & 14 almonds

<table>
<tr><td colspan="4">

Rest & Active Recovery Blueprint

Protein: 35 blocks

Veggies: 7.5 blocks

Fats: 7.5 blocks

</td></tr>
</table>

REST DAYS – 280 lbs.

The weight loss formula for rest and active recovery days includes healthy proteins, vegetables, and essential fats. We want to eliminate all sugars and starches on rest days as your body will not need them.

4 Meals Menu Plan

Macro	Meal 1	Meal 2	Meal 3	Meal 4	Total
Protein	8	10	8	9	35
Veggie	2	2	2	1 ½	7 ½
Fat	2	1 ½	2	2	7 ½

5 Meals Menu Plan

Macro	Meal 1	Meal 2	Meal 3	Meal 4	Meal 5	Total
Protein	5	6	7	9 ½	7 ½	35
Veggie	2	1 ½	1	2	1	7 ½
Fat	1 ½	1	1	2	2	7 ½

6 Meals Menu Plan

Macro	Meal 1	Meal 2	Meal 3	Meal 4	Meal 5	Meal 6	Total
Protein	4	4 ½	9	5	7	5 ½	35
Veggie	1	1	1 ½	1	2	1	7 ½
Fat	1	1	1	1	1 ½	2	7 ½

Following are example menus for the weight loss formula covering rest and active recovery days for those in the 280 pound category. You may look at the Meal Chart to pick different foods that suit your taste buds.

Example Menus

Rest & Recovery Days

280 lbs.

4 Meals Plan

Breakfast: Omelette made w/1 whole Omega-3 egg, 5 egg whites, 5 oz. beef slices, 1 cup sliced red bell pepper, ¼ cup chopped onions & ½ cup chopped tomatoes - cooked in 2 tsp. EVOO; 1 cup green tea

Lunch: 10 oz. grilled chicken breast & ¾ cup baked zucchini & 9 cherry tomatoes drizzled with 1-½ tsp. EVOO on top

Dinner: 12 oz. baked tilapia & 16 spears asparagus rolled in 2 tsp. coconut oil

Bedtime Snack: Cereal made with 1 cup low-fat cottage cheese, 1-⅔ scoops low-carb vanilla protein powder, and 2 Tbs. chia seeds; ¾ cup raw broccoli & 6 large baby carrots

5 Meals Plan

Breakfast: Scrambled 1 whole Omega-3 egg, 5 egg whites with 1-½ cups raw mushroom and ¼ cup chopped onions & topped with ½ oz. Mozzarella cheese; 4 slices turkey bacon; ½ cup low-sodium V-8; 1 cup green tea

Lunch: 9 oz. tuna mixed with 1 Tbs. EVOO mayo on top of Romaine lettuce, ½ cup tomatoes, 1 cup cucumbers & ¼ cup onions

Snack: Protein shake made with 2-⅓ scoops low-carb protein powder; 6 large baby carrots; 2 Brazil nut

Dinner: 9.5 oz. grilled flank steak; 1 cup steamed broccoli drizzled with 2 tsp. flaxseed oil

Bedtime Snack: 1 cup Greek yogurt mixed with 1.5 scoops low-carb vanilla protein powder; 6 cherry tomatoes; 2 Tbs. almonds

6 Meals Plan

Breakfast: Omelette w/4 egg whites, 4 turkey bacon, ¼ cup onions & ½ cup sweet bell pepper; ¼ cup avocado slices; 1 c. green tea

Snack: 1-½ cup tofu fried in 1 tsp. EVOO; 1 cup raw slices of red bell pepper

Lunch: 9 oz. turkey breast chunks on top of baby spinach & 9 cherry tomatoes drizzled with 1 tsp. flax oil

Snack: 7.5 oz. tuna mixed with 1 Tbs. EVOO mayo & served with ¾ cup raw broccoli flowerets & 3 baby carrots

Dinner: 10.5 oz. salmon & coleslaw made with ¾ cup shredded cabbage, 2 small carrot stick & 1.5 Tbs. EVOO mayo

Bedtime Snack: 1-¾ scoops low-carb protein powder (shake), 6 large baby carrots & 14 almonds

9 – Blueprints & Examples for Normal Workout Days

What are normal workout days?

✓ Normal workout days include any form of exercise that raises your heart rate for an extended period of time – at least 20 to 60 minutes.

✓ Normal workout days may include the following exercises: any form of cardio, high intensity interval training, jump roping, hiking, kickboxing, weight training, and more.

✓ On an intensity scale of 1 to 10, where 1 equates to no effort and 10 equate to all-out effort, a normal intensity level would be 5 to 8.

✓ All workouts will be included as a normal workout day, other than the one or two most strenuous workout days of the week, as well as rest and activity recovery days.

When to Use this Blueprint

All workouts during the week will be considered normal workout days, other than the one or two most strenuous workout days, as well as rest and activity recovery days. The blueprint for normal workout days should be the most widely used which means that you should be getting some form of exercise in most days as discussed in Chapter 7.

What Foods this Blueprint Includes

A few extra calories are added for the extra energy your body will need on normal workout and cardio days, but only enough to still allow you to burn body fat. Proteins are included to nourish your body, keep you satiated, preserve lean muscle mass, and keep your metabolism on fire. Vegetable carbohydrates are built in to supply your body with vitamins, minerals, and phytonutrients. Vegetables will also protect your body from damaging free radicals by providing it with antioxidants. The fiber in vegetables will help rid your body of metabolic waste. A small portion of fruit carbohydrates are included to replenish your muscles and brain with energy that was depleted during normal workouts – but just enough to not be stored as body fat. Dietary fats will balance out your meals and will help supply you with essential nutrients for every cell in your body to function optimally. You should exclude fats in your post-workout meal. Lentil, whole grain, and tuber carbohydrates are eliminated as your body will not need the extra sugars or starches on normal workout or cardio days. This will also help you burn body fat faster.

How to Count Blocks of Food

An example of counting blocks of food has been given in Chapter 7. However, a new example detailing this particular blueprint has been given below.

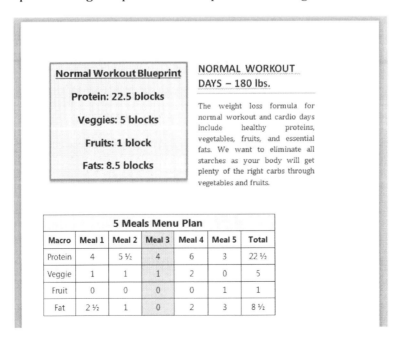

For this component of Phase 3 nutrition planning, you have the option of choosing from five or six meals per day. The example just given shows the "5 Meals Menu Plan." At the top of each page, you will see the blocks of food allotted for this weight category. There are 22.5 protein blocks, 5 veggie blocks, 1 fruit block, and 8.5 fat blocks for the "5 Meals Menu Plan" of the 180 pound menu plan. The meal shaded in gray (Meal 3) is your post workout meal where dietary fat is excluded. On the opposite page, you will be given examples for each menu plan as shown below.

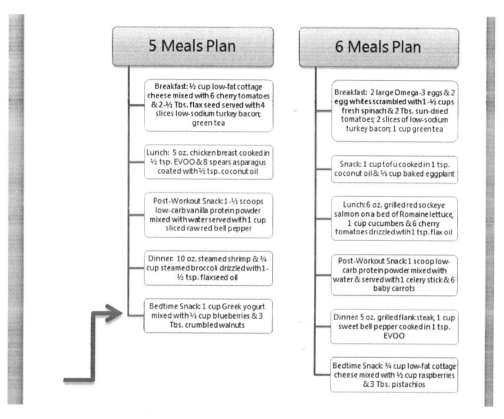

On the 180 pound menu plan, you will see how many blocks are allotted for each meal. Look at Meal 5. It includes 3 protein blocks, 0 vegetable blocks, 1 fruit block, and 3 fat blocks. If you then look at the bedtime snack meal example for the "5 Meals Plan" above, you will see that that it consists of one cup of Greek yogurt (3 proteins), ⅓ cup blueberries (1 fruit), and two tablespoons of crumbled walnuts (2 fats). The foods selected are taken from the meal charts in Chapter 12 to find the serving size of each food by using the block number given on the menu plan multiplied by the serving size given on the meal charts. You may refer to Chapter 7 to determine correct calculations.

Normal Workout Blueprint
Protein: 15 blocks
Veggies: 3 blocks
Fruits: 1 block
Fats: 5.5 blocks

The weight loss formula for normal workout and cardio days includes healthy proteins, vegetables, fruits, and essential fats. We want to eliminate all starches as your body will get plenty of the right carbs through vegetables and fruits.

5 Meals Menu Plan

Macro	Meal 1	Meal 2	Meal 3	Meal 4	Meal 5	Total
Protein	3	3	3	3	3	15
Veggie	1	½	½	1	0	3
Fruit	0	0	0	0	1	1
Fat	1	1	0	1	2 ½	5 ½

6 Meals Menu Plan

Macro	Meal 1	Meal 2	Meal 3	Meal 4	Meal 5	Meal 6	Total
Protein	2 ½	2 ½	2 ½	2 ½	2 ½	2 ½	15
Veggie	½	½	½	½	1	0	3
Fruit	0	0	0	0	0	1	1
Fat	1	½	1	0	1	2	5 ½

Following are example menus for the weight loss formula covering normal workout and cardio days for those in the 120 pound category. You may look at the Meal Chart to pick different foods that suit your taste buds.

Example Menus

Normal Workout Days

120 lbs.

5 Meals Plan

Breakfast: ¾ cup low-fat cottage cheese mixed with 6 cherry tomatoes & 1 Tbs. flax seed; green tea

Lunch: 3 oz. chicken breast cooked in ½ tsp. EVOO & 4 spears asparagus coated with ½ tsp. coconut oil

Post-Workout Snack: 1 scoop low-carb vanilla protein powder mixed with water & served with ½ cup sliced raw red bell pepper

Dinner: 6 oz. steamed shrimp & ½ cup steamed broccoli drizzled with 1 tsp. flaxseed oil

Bedtime Snack: 1 cup Greek yogurt mixed with ⅓ cup blueberries & 2-½ Tbs. crumbled walnuts

6 Meals Plan

Breakfast: 1 large Omega-3 eggs & 3 egg whites scrambled with 1-½ cups fresh spinach & 1 Tbs. sun-dried tomato; 1 slice of low-sodium turkey bacon; 1 cup green tea

Snack: ¾ cup tofu cooked in ½ tsp. coconut oil & ⅓ cup baked eggplant

Lunch: 3-¾ oz. grilled red sockeye salmon on a bed of Romaine lettuce & 1 cup cucumbers drizzled wtih 1 tsp. flax oil

Post-Workout Snack: ¾ scoop low-carb protein powder mixed with water & served with 1 celery stick & 3 baby carrots

Dinner: 2-½ oz. grilled flank steak, 1 cup sweet bell pepper cooked in 1 tsp. EVOO

Bedtime Snack: ⅔ cup low-fat cottage cheese mixed with ½ cup raspberries & 2 Tbs. pistachios

Normal Workout Blueprint

Protein: 16 blocks

Veggies: 3 blocks

Fruits: 1 block

Fats: 6 blocks

NORMAL WORKOUT DAYS – 130 lbs.

The weight loss formula for normal workout and cardio days includes healthy proteins, vegetables, fruits, and essential fats. We want to eliminate all starches as your body will get plenty of the right carbs through vegetables and fruits.

5 Meals Menu Plan

Macro	Meal 1	Meal 2	Meal 3	Meal 4	Meal 5	Total
Protein	3	3	3	4	3	16
Veggie	1	½	½	1	0	3
Fruit	0	0	0	0	1	1
Fat	1	1	0	1	3	6

6 Meals Menu Plan

Macro	Meal 1	Meal 2	Meal 3	Meal 4	Meal 5	Meal 6	Total
Protein	2 ½	2 ½	2 ½	2 ½	3	3	16
Veggie	½	½	½	½	1	0	3
Fruit	0	0	0	0	0	1	1
Fat	1	1	1	0	1	2	6

Following are example menus for the weight loss formula covering normal workout and cardio days for those in the 130 pound category. You may look at the Meal Chart to pick different foods that suit your taste buds.

Example Menus

Normal Workout Days

130 lbs.

5 Meals Plan

Breakfast: ¾ cup low-fat cottage cheese mixed with 6 cherry tomatoes & 1 Tbs. flax seed; green tea

Lunch: 3 oz. chicken breast cooked in ½ tsp. EVOO & 4 spears asparagus coated with ½ tsp. coconut oil

Post-Workout Snack: 1 scoop low-carb vanilla protein powder mixed with water & served with ½ cup sliced raw red bell pepper

Dinner: 8 oz. steamed shrimp & ½ cup steamed broccoli drizzled with 1 tsp. flaxseed oil

Bedtime Snack: 1 cup Greek yogurt mixed with ⅓ cup blueberries & 3 Tbs. crumbled walnuts

6 Meals Plan

Breakfast: 1 large Omega-3 eggs & 3 egg whites scrambled with 1-½ cups fresh spinach & 1 Tbs. sun-dried tomato; 1 slice of low-sodium turkey bacon; 1 cup green tea

Snack: ¾ cup tofu cooked in 1 tsp. coconut oil & ⅓ cup baked eggplant

Lunch: 3-¾ oz. grilled red sockeye salmon on a bed of Romaine lettuce & 1 cup cucumbers drizzled wtih 1 tsp. flax oil

Post-Workout Snack: ¾ scoop low-carb protein powder mixed with water & served with 1 celery stick & 3 baby carrots

Dinner: 3 oz. grilled flank steak, 1 cup sweet bell pepper cooked in 1 tsp. EVOO

Bedtime Snack: ¾ cup low-fat cottage cheese mixed with ½ cup raspberries & 2 Tbs. pistachios

Normal Workout Blueprint

Protein: 17.5 blocks

Veggies: 3.5 blocks

Fruits: 1 block

Fats: 6.5 blocks

NORMAL WORKOUT DAYS – 140 lbs.

The weight loss formula for normal workout and cardio days includes healthy proteins, vegetables, fruits, and essential fats. We want to eliminate all starches as your body will get plenty of the right carbs through vegetables and fruits.

5 Meals Menu Plan

Macro	Meal 1	Meal 2	Meal 3	Meal 4	Meal 5	Total
Protein	3 ½	3	3 ½	4	3 ½	17 ½
Veggie	1	½	1	1	0	3 ½
Fruit	0	0	0	0	1	1
Fat	1	1	0	1 ½	3	6 ½

6 Meals Menu Plan

Macro	Meal 1	Meal 2	Meal 3	Meal 4	Meal 5	Meal 6	Total
Protein	3	2 ½	3	3	3	3	17 ½
Veggie	½	½	1	½	1	0	3 ½
Fruit	0	0	0	0	0	1	1
Fat	1	1	1	0	1	2 ½	6 ½

Following are example menus for the weight loss formula covering normal workout and cardio days for those in the 140 pound category. You may look at the Meal Chart to pick different foods that suit your taste buds.

Example Menus

Normal Workout Days

140 lbs.

5 Meals Plan

Breakfast: ½ cup low-fat cottage cheese mixed with 6 cherry tomatoes & 1 Tbs. flax seed served with 3 slices low-sodium turkey bacon; green tea

Lunch: 3 oz. chicken breast cooked in ½ tsp. EVOO & 4 spears asparagus coated with ½ tsp. coconut oil

Post-Workout Snack: 1 heaping scoop low-carb vanilla protein powder mxied with water & served with 1 cup sliced raw red bell pepper

Dinner: 8 oz. steamed shrimp & ½ cup steamed broccoli drizzled with 1-½ tsp. flaxseed oil

Bedtime Snack: 1 heaping cup Greek yogurt mixed with ⅓ cup blueberries & 3 Tbs. crumbled walnuts

6 Meals Plan

Breakfast: 1 large Omega-3 eggs & 3 egg whites scrambled with 1-½ cups fresh spinach, & 1 Tbs. sun-dried tomato; 2 slices of low-sodium turkey bacon; 1 cup green tea

Snack: ¾ cup tofu cooked in 1 tsp. coconut oil & ⅓ cup baked eggplant

Lunch: 4-½ oz. grilled red sockeye salmon on a bed of Romaine lettuce, 1 cup cucumbers & 6 cherry tomatoes drizzled wtih 1 tsp. flax oil

Post-Workout Snack: 1 scoop low-carb protein powder mixed with water & served with 1 celery stick & 3 baby carrots

Dinner: 3 oz. grilled flank steak, 1 cup sweet bell pepper cooked in 1 tsp. EVOO

Bedtime Snack: ¾ cup low-fat cottage cheese mixed with ½ cup raspberries & 2-½ Tbs. pistachios

<table>
<tr><td colspan="2">

Normal Workout Blueprint

Protein: 19 blocks

Veggies: 4 blocks

Fruits: 1 block

Fats: 7 blocks
</td></tr>
</table>

NORMAL WORKOUT DAYS – 150 lbs.

The weight loss formula for normal workout and cardio days includes healthy proteins, vegetables, fruits, and essential fats. We want to eliminate all starches as your body will get plenty of the right carbs through vegetables and fruits.

5 Meals Menu Plan

Macro	Meal 1	Meal 2	Meal 3	Meal 4	Meal 5	Total
Protein	4	4	4	4	3	19
Veggie	1	1	1	1	0	4
Fruit	0	0	0	0	1	1
Fat	2	1	0	1	3	7

6 Meals Menu Plan

Macro	Meal 1	Meal 2	Meal 3	Meal 4	Meal 5	Meal 6	Total
Protein	3	3	3	3	4	3	19
Veggie	1	½	1	½	1	0	4
Fruit	0	0	0	0	0	1	1
Fat	1	1	1	0	1	3	7

Following are example menus for the weight loss formula covering normal workout and cardio days for those in the 150 pound category. You may look at the Meal Chart to pick different foods that suit your taste buds.

Example Menus

Normal Workout Days

150 lbs.

5 Meals Plan

Breakfast: ½ cup low-fat cottage cheese mixed with 6 cherry tomatoes & 2 Tbs. flax seed served with 4 slices low-sodium turkey bacon; green tea

Lunch: 4 oz. chicken breast cooked in ½ tsp. EVOO & 8 spears asparagus coated with ½ tsp. coconut oil

Post-Workout Snack: 1-⅓ scoops low-carb vanilla protein powder mixed with water & served with 1 cup sliced raw red bell pepper

Dinner: 8 oz. steamed shrimp & ½ cup steamed broccoli drizzled with 1 tsp. flaxseed oil

Bedtime Snack: 1 cup Greek yogurt mixed with ⅓ cup blueberries & 3 Tbs. crumbled walnuts

6 Meals Plan

Breakfast: 1 large Omega-3 eggs & 3 egg whites scrambled with 1-½ cups fresh spinach & 2 Tbs. sun-dried tomatoes; 2 slices of low-sodium turkey bacon; 1 cup green tea

Snack: 1 cup tofu cooked in 1 tsp. coconut oil & ⅓ cup baked eggplant

Lunch: 4-½ oz. grilled red sockeye salmon on a bed of Romaine lettuce, 1 cup cucumbers & 6 cherry tomatoes drizzled wtih 1 tsp. flax oil

Post-Workout Snack: 1 scoop low-carb protein powder mixed with water & served with 1 celery stick & 3 baby carrots

Dinner: 4 oz. grilled flank steak, 1 cup sweet bell pepper cooked in 1 tsp. EVOO

Bedtime Snack: ¾ cup low-fat cottage cheese mixed with ½ cup raspberries & 3 Tbs. pistachios

Normal Workout Blueprint	NORMAL WORKOUT DAYS – 160 lbs.

Normal Workout Blueprint

Protein: 20 blocks

Veggies: 4 blocks

Fruits: 1 block

Fats: 7.5 blocks

NORMAL WORKOUT DAYS – 160 lbs.

The weight loss formula for normal workout and cardio days includes healthy proteins, vegetables, fruits, and essential fats. We want to eliminate all starches as your body will get plenty of the right carbs through vegetables and fruits.

5 Meals Menu Plan

Macro	Meal 1	Meal 2	Meal 3	Meal 4	Meal 5	Total
Protein	4	4	4	5	3	20
Veggie	1	1	1	1	0	4
Fruit	0	0	0	0	1	1
Fat	2	1	0	1 ½	3	7 ½

6 Meals Menu Plan

Macro	Meal 1	Meal 2	Meal 3	Meal 4	Meal 5	Meal 6	Total
Protein	3	3	4	3	4	3	20
Veggie	1	½	1	½	1	0	4
Fruit	0	0	0	0	0	1	1
Fat	1	1	1	0	2	2 ½	7 ½

Following are example menus for the weight loss formula covering normal workout and cardio days for those in the 160 pound category. You may look at the Meal Chart to pick different foods that suit your taste buds.

Example Menus

Normal Workout Days

160 lbs.

5 Meals Plan

Breakfast: ½ cup low-fat cottage cheese mixed with 6 cherry tomatoes & 2 Tbs. flax seed served with 4 slices low-sodium turkey bacon; green tea

Lunch: 4 oz. chicken breast cooked in ½ tsp. EVOO & 8 spears asparagus coated with ½ tsp. coconut oil

Post-Workout Snack: 1-⅓ scoops low-carb vanilla protein powder mixed with water & served with 1 cup sliced raw red bell pepper

Dinner: 10 oz. steamed shrimp & ½ cup steamed broccoli drizzled with 1-½ tsp. flaxseed oil

Bedtime Snack: 1 cup Greek yogurt mixed with ⅓ cup blueberries & 3 Tbs. crumbled walnuts

6 Meals Plan

Breakfast: 1 large Omega-3 eggs & 3 egg whites scrambled with 1-½ cups fresh spinach & 2 Tbs. sun-dried tomatoes; 2 slices of low-sodium turkey bacon; 1 cup green tea

Snack: 1 cup tofu cooked in 1 tsp. coconut oil & ⅓ cup baked eggplant

Lunch: 6 oz. grilled red sockeye salmon on a bed of Romaine lettuce, 1 cup cucumbers & 6 cherry tomatoes drizzled wtih 1 tsp. flax oil

Post-Workout Snack: 1 scoop low-carb protein powder mixed with water & served with 1 celery stick & 3 baby carrots

Dinner: 4 oz. grilled flank steak, 1 cup sweet bell pepper cooked in 2 tsp. EVOO

Bedtime Snack: ¾ cup low-fat cottage cheese mixed with ½ cup raspberries & 2-½ Tbs. pistachios

Normal Workout Blueprint

Protein: 21 blocks

Veggies: 4.5 blocks

Fruits: 1 block

Fats: 8 blocks

NORMAL WORKOUT DAYS – 170 lbs.

The weight loss formula for normal workout and cardio days includes healthy proteins, vegetables, fruits, and essential fats. We want to eliminate all starches as your body will get plenty of the right carbs through vegetables and fruits.

5 Meals Menu Plan

Macro	Meal 1	Meal 2	Meal 3	Meal 4	Meal 5	Total
Protein	4	5	4	5	3	21
Veggie	1	1	1	1 ½	0	4 ½
Fruit	0	0	0	0	1	1
Fat	2 ½	1	0	1 ½	3	8

6 Meals Menu Plan

Macro	Meal 1	Meal 2	Meal 3	Meal 4	Meal 5	Meal 6	Total
Protein	3	3	4	3	5	3	21
Veggie	1	½	1	1	1	0	4 ½
Fruit	0	0	0	0	0	1	1
Fat	2	1	1	0	1	3	8

Following are example menus for the weight loss formula covering normal workout and cardio days for those in the 170 pound category. You may look at the Meal Chart to pick different foods that suit your taste buds.

Example Menus

Normal Workout Days

170 lbs.

5 Meals Plan

Breakfast: ½ cup low-fat cottage cheese mixed with 6 cherry tomatoes & 2-½ Tbs. flax seed served with 4 slices low-sodium turkey bacon; green tea

Lunch: 5 oz. chicken breast cooked in ½ tsp. EVOO & 8 spears asparagus coated with ½ tsp. coconut oil

Post-Workout Snack: 1-⅓ scoops low-carb vanilla protein powder mixed with water served with 1 cup sliced raw red bell pepper

Dinner: 10 oz. steamed shrimp & ¾ cup steamed broccoli drizzled with 1-½ tsp. flaxseed oil

Bedtime Snack: 1 cup Greek yogurt mixed with ⅓ cup blueberries & 3 Tbs. crumbled walnuts

6 Meals Plan

Breakfast: 2 large Omega-3 eggs & 2 egg whites scrambled with 1-½ cups fresh spinach & 2 Tbs. sun-dried tomatoes; 2 slices of low-sodium turkey bacon; 1 cup green tea

Snack: 1 cup tofu cooked in 1 tsp. coconut oil & ⅓ cup baked eggplant

Lunch: 6 oz. grilled red sockeye salmon on a bed of Romaine lettuce, 1 cup cucumbers & 6 cherry tomatoes drizzled wtih 1 tsp. flax oil

Post-Workout Snack: 1 scoop low-carb protein powder mixed with water & served with 1 celery stick & 6 baby carrots

Dinner: 5 oz. grilled flank steak, 1 cup sweet bell pepper cooked in 1 tsp. EVOO

Bedtime Snack: ¾ cup low-fat cottage cheese mixed with ½ cup raspberries & 3 Tbs. pistachios

Normal Workout Blueprint

Protein: 22.5 blocks

Veggies: 5 blocks

Fruits: 1 block

Fats: 8.5 blocks

NORMAL WORKOUT DAYS – 180 lbs.

The weight loss formula for normal workout and cardio days includes healthy proteins, vegetables, fruits, and essential fats. We want to eliminate all starches as your body will get plenty of the right carbs through vegetables and fruits.

5 Meals Menu Plan

Macro	Meal 1	Meal 2	Meal 3	Meal 4	Meal 5	Total
Protein	4	5 ½	4	6	3	22 ½
Veggie	1	1	1	2	0	5
Fruit	0	0	0	0	1	1
Fat	2 ½	1	0	2	3	8 ½

6 Meals Menu Plan

Macro	Meal 1	Meal 2	Meal 3	Meal 4	Meal 5	Meal 6	Total
Protein	3 ½	3	4	4	5	3	22 ½
Veggie	1	1	1	1	1	0	5
Fruit	0	0	0	0	0	1	1
Fat	2	1	1	0	1 ½	3	8 ½

Following are example menus for the weight loss formula covering normal workout and cardio days for those in the 180 pound category. You may look at the Meal Chart to pick different foods that suit your taste buds.

Example Menus

Normal Workout Days

180 lbs.

5 Meals Plan

Breakfast: ½ cup low-fat cottage cheese mixed with 6 cherry tomatoes & 2-½ Tbs. flax seed served with 4 slices low-sodium turkey bacon; green tea

Lunch: 5-½ oz. chicken breast cooked in ½ tsp. EVOO & 8 spears asparagus coated with ½ tsp. coconut oil

Post-Workout Snack: 1-⅓ scoops low-carb vanilla protein powder mixed with water and served with 1 cup sliced raw red bell pepper

Dinner: 12 oz. steamed shrimp & 1 cup steamed broccoli drizzled with 2 tsp. flaxseed oil

Bedtime Snack: 1 cup Greek yogurt mixed with ⅓ cup blueberries & 3 Tbs. crumbled walnuts

6 Meals Plan

Breakfast: 2 large Omega-3 eggs & 2 egg whites scrambled with 1-½ cups fresh spinach & 2 Tbs. sun-dried tomatoes; 3 slices of low-sodium turkey bacon; 1 cup green tea

Snack: 1 cup tofu cooked in 1 tsp. coconut oil & ¾ cup baked eggplant

Lunch: 6 oz. grilled red sockeye salmon on a bed of Romaine lettuce, 1 cup cucumbers & 6 cherry tomatoes drizzled wtih 1 tsp. flax oil

Post-Workout Snack: 1-⅓ scoop low-carb protein powder mixed with water & served with 1 celery stick & 6 baby carrots

Dinner: 5 oz. grilled flank steak, 1 cup sweet bell pepper cooked in 1-½ tsp. EVOO

Bedtime Snack: ¾ cup low-fat cottage cheese mixed with ½ cup raspberries & 3 Tbs. pistachios

Normal Workout Blueprint

Protein: 24 blocks

Veggies: 5 blocks

Fruits: 1 block

Fats: 9 blocks

NORMAL WORKOUT DAYS – 190 lbs.

The weight loss formula for normal workout and cardio days includes healthy proteins, vegetables, fruits, and essential fats. We want to eliminate all starches as your body will get plenty of the right carbs through vegetables and fruits.

5 Meals Menu Plan

Macro	Meal 1	Meal 2	Meal 3	Meal 4	Meal 5	Total
Protein	4	6	4	7	3	24
Veggie	1	1	1	2	0	5
Fruit	0	0	0	0	1	1
Fat	2	2	0	2	3	9

6 Meals Menu Plan

Macro	Meal 1	Meal 2	Meal 3	Meal 4	Meal 5	Meal 6	Total
Protein	4	3	4	4	6	3	24
Veggie	1	1	1	1	1	0	5
Fruit	0	0	0	0	0	1	1
Fat	2	1	1	0	2	3	9

Following are example menus for the weight loss formula covering normal workout and cardio days for those in the 190 pound category. You may look at the Meal Chart to pick different foods that suit your taste buds.

Example Menus

Normal Workout Days

190 lbs.

5 Meals Plan

Breakfast: ½ cup low-fat cottage cheese mixed with 6 cherry tomatoes & 2 Tbs. flax seed served with 4 slices low-sodium turkey bacon; green tea

Lunch: 6 oz. chicken breast cooked in 1 tsp. EVOO & 8 spears asparagus coated with 1 tsp. coconut oil

Post-Workout Snack: 1-⅓ scoops low-carb vanilla protein powder mixed with water and served with 1 cup sliced raw red bell pepper

Dinner: 4 oz. lean steak & 6 oz. steamed shrimp & 1 cup steamed broccoli drizzled with 2 tsp. flaxseed oil

Bedtime Snack: 1 cup Greek yogurt mixed with ⅓ cup blueberries & 3 Tbs. crumbled walnuts

6 Meals Plan

Breakfast: 2 large Omega-3 eggs & 2 egg whites scrambled with 1-½ cups fresh spinach & 2 Tbs. sun-dried tomatoes; 4 slices of low-sodium turkey bacon; 1 cup green tea

Snack: 1 cup tofu cooked in 1 tsp. coconut oil & ¾ cup baked eggplant

Lunch: 6 oz. grilled red sockeye salmon on a bed of Romaine lettuce, 1 cup cucumbers & 6 cherry tomatoes drizzled wtih 1 tsp. flax oil

Post-Workout Snack: 1-⅓ scoop low-carb protein powder mixed with water & served with 1 celery stick & 6 baby carrots

Dinner: 6 oz. grilled flank steak, 1 cup sweet bell pepper cooked in 2 tsp. EVOO

Bedtime Snack: ¾ cup low-fat cottage cheese mixed with ½ cup raspberries & 3 Tbs. pistachios

Normal Workout Blueprint

Protein: 25 blocks

Veggies: 5.5 blocks

Fruits: 1 block

Fats: 9.5 blocks

NORMAL WORKOUT DAYS – 200 lbs.

The weight loss formula for normal workout and cardio days includes healthy proteins, vegetables, fruits, and essential fats. We want to eliminate all starches as your body will get plenty of the right carbs through vegetables and fruits.

5 Meals Menu Plan

Macro	Meal 1	Meal 2	Meal 3	Meal 4	Meal 5	Total
Protein	4	7	4	7	3	25
Veggie	1 ½	1	1	2	0	5 ½
Fruit	0	0	0	0	1	1
Fat	2	2	0	2 ½	3	9 ½

6 Meals Menu Plan

Macro	Meal 1	Meal 2	Meal 3	Meal 4	Meal 5	Meal 6	Total
Protein	4	3	5	4	6	3	25
Veggie	1	1	1	1	1 ½	0	5 ½
Fruit	0	0	0	0	0	1	1
Fat	2	1 ½	1	0	2	3	9 ½

Following are example menus for the weight loss formula covering normal workout and cardio days for those in the 200 pound category. You may look at the Meal Chart to pick different foods that suit your taste buds.

Example Menus

Normal Workout Days

200 lbs.

5 Meals Plan

Breakfast: ½ cup low-fat cottage cheese mixed with 9 cherry tomatoes & 2 Tbs. flax seed served with 4 slices low-sodium turkey bacon; green tea

Lunch: 7 oz. chicken breast cooked in 1 tsp. EVOO & 8 spears asparagus coated with 1 tsp. coconut oil

Post-Workout Snack: 1-⅓ scoops low-carb vanilla protein powder mixed with water and served with 1 cup sliced raw red bell pepper

Dinner: 4 oz. lean steak & 6 oz. steamed shrimp & 1 cup steamed broccoli drizzled with 2-½ tsp. flaxseed oil

Bedtime Snack: 1 cup Greek yogurt mixed with ⅓ cup blueberries & 3 Tbs. crumbled walnuts

6 Meals Plan

Breakfast: 2 large Omega-3 eggs & 2 egg whites scrambled with 1-½ cups fresh spinach & 2 Tbs. sun-dried tomatoes, 4 slices of low-sodium turkey bacon; 1 cup green tea

Snack: 1 cup tofu cooked in 1-½ tsp. coconut oil & ¾ cup baked eggplant

Lunch: 7-½ oz. grilled red sockeye salmon on a bed of Romaine lettuce, 1 cup cucumbers & 6 cherry tomatoes drizzled wtih 1 tsp. flax oil

Post-Workout Snack: 1-⅓ scoop low-carb protein powder mixed with water & served with 1 celery stick & 6 baby carrots

Dinner: 6 oz. grilled flank steak, 1 cup sweet bell pepper & ¼ cup chopped onions cooked in 2 tsp. EVOO

Bedtime Snack: ¾ cup low-fat cottage cheese mixed with ½ cup raspberries & 3 Tbs. pistachios

Normal Workout Blueprint

Protein: 26 blocks

Veggies: 6 blocks

Fruits: 1 block

Fats: 10 blocks

NORMAL WORKOUT DAYS – 210 lbs.

The weight loss formula for normal workout and cardio days includes healthy proteins, vegetables, fruits, and essential fats. We want to eliminate all starches as your body will get plenty of the right carbs through vegetables and fruits.

5 Meals Menu Plan

Macro	Meal 1	Meal 2	Meal 3	Meal 4	Meal 5	Total
Protein	4	7	4	8	3	26
Veggie	2	1	1	2	0	6
Fruit	0	0	0	0	1	1
Fat	2	2	0	3	3	10

6 Meals Menu Plan

Macro	Meal 1	Meal 2	Meal 3	Meal 4	Meal 5	Meal 6	Total
Protein	4	3	5	4	7	3	26
Veggie	1	1	1	1	2	0	6
Fruit	0	0	0	0	0	1	1
Fat	2	2	1	0	2	3	10

Following are example menus for the weight loss formula covering normal workout and cardio days for those in the 210 pound category. You may look at the Meal Chart to pick different foods that suit your taste buds.

Example Menus

Normal Workout Days

210 lbs.

5 Meals Plan

Breakfast: ½ cup low-fat cottage cheese mixed with 6 cherry tomatoes, 1 cup cubed cucumbers & 2 Tbs. flax seed served with 4 slices low-sodium turkey bacon; ½ cup low-sodium V-8 juice & green tea

Lunch: 7 oz. chicken breast cooked in 1 tsp. EVOO & 8 spears asparagus coated with 1 tsp. coconut oil

Post-Workout Snack: 1-⅓ scoops low-carb vanilla protein powder mixed with water served with 1 cup sliced raw red bell pepper

Dinner: 5 oz. lean steak & 6 oz. steamed shrimp & 1 cup steamed broccoli drizzled with 1 Tbs. flaxseed oil

Bedtime Snack: 1 cup Greek yogurt mixed with ⅓ cup blueberries & 3 Tbs. crumbled walnuts

6 Meals Plan

Breakfast: 2 large Omega-3 eggs & 2 egg whites scrambled with 1-½ cups fresh spinach & 2 Tbs. sun-dried tomatoes, 4 slices of low-sodium turkey bacon; 1 cup green tea

Snack: 1 cup tofu cooked in 2 tsp. coconut oil & ¾ cup baked eggplant

Lunch: 7-½ oz. grilled red sockeye salmon on a bed of Romaine lettuce, 1 cup cucumbers & 6 cherry tomatoes drizzled wtih 1 tsp. flax oil

Post-Workout Snack: 1-⅓ scoop low-carb protein powder mixed with water & served with 1 celery stick & 6 baby carrots

Dinner: 7 oz. grilled flank steak, 1 cup sweet bell pepper & ½ cup chopped onions cooked in 2 tsp. EVOO

Bedtime Snack: ¾ cup low-fat cottage cheese mixed with ½ cup raspberries & 3 Tbs. pistachios

Normal Workout Blueprint	NORMAL WORKOUT DAYS – 220 lbs.

Normal Workout Blueprint

Protein: 27.5 blocks

Veggies: 6 blocks

Fruits: 1 block

Fats: 10 blocks

NORMAL WORKOUT DAYS – 220 lbs.

The weight loss formula for normal workout and cardio days includes healthy proteins, vegetables, fruits, and essential fats. We want to eliminate all starches as your body will get plenty of the right carbs through vegetables and fruits.

5 Meals Menu Plan

Macro	Meal 1	Meal 2	Meal 3	Meal 4	Meal 5	Total
Protein	4 ½	7	5	8	3	27 ½
Veggie	2	1	1	2	0	6
Fruit	0	0	0	0	1	1
Fat	2	2	0	2	4	10

6 Meals Menu Plan

Macro	Meal 1	Meal 2	Meal 3	Meal 4	Meal 5	Meal 6	Total
Protein	4	3	6	4	7 ½	3	27 ½
Veggie	1	1	1	1	2	0	6
Fruit	0	0	0	0	0	1	1
Fat	2	2	1	0	2	3	10

Following are example menus for the weight loss formula covering normal workout and cardio days for those in the 220 pound category. You may look at the Meal Chart to pick different foods that suit your taste buds.

Example Menus

Normal Workout Days

220 lbs.

5 Meals Plan

Breakfast: ½ cup low-fat cottage cheese mixed with 6 cherry tomatoes, 1 cup cubed cucumbers & 2-½ Tbs. flax seed served with 5 slices low-sodium turkey bacon; ½ cup low-sodium V-8 juice & green tea

Lunch: 7 oz. chicken breast cooked in 1 tsp. EVOO & 8 spears asparagus coated with 1 tsp. coconut oil

Post-Workout Snack: 1-⅔ scoops low-carb vanilla protein powder mixed with water and served with 1 cup sliced raw red bell pepper

Dinner: 5 oz. lean steak & 6 oz. steamed shrimp & 1 cup steamed broccoli drizzled with 2 tsp. flaxseed oil

Bedtime Snack: 1 cup Greek yogurt mixed with ⅓ cup blueberries & 4 Tbs. crumbled walnuts

6 Meals Plan

Breakfast: 2 large Omega-3 eggs & 2 egg whites scrambled with 1-½ cups fresh spinach & 2 Tbs. sun-dried tomatoes, 4 slices of low-sodium turkey bacon; 1 cup green tea

Snack: 1 cup tofu cooked in 2 tsp. coconut oil & ¾ cup baked eggplant

Lunch: 9 oz. grilled red sockeye salmon on a bed of Romaine lettuce, 1 cup cucumbers & 6 cherry tomatoes drizzled wtih 1 tsp. flax oil

Post-Workout Snack: 1-⅓ scoop low-carb protein powder mixed with water served with 1 celery stick & 6 baby carrots

Dinner: 7-½ oz. grilled flank steak, 1 cup sweet bell pepper & ½ cup chopped onions cooked in 1-½ tsp. EVOO

Bedtime Snack: ¾ cup low-fat cottage cheese mixed with ½ cup raspberries & 3 Tbs. pistachios

Normal Workout Blueprint

Protein: 29 blocks

Veggies: 6.5 blocks

Fruits: 1 block

Fats: 10.5 blocks

NORMAL WORKOUT DAYS – 230 lbs.

The weight loss formula for normal workout and cardio days includes healthy proteins, vegetables, fruits, and essential fats. We want to eliminate all starches as your body will get plenty of the right carbs through vegetables and fruits.

5 Meals Menu Plan

Macro	Meal 1	Meal 2	Meal 3	Meal 4	Meal 5	Total
Protein	5	8	5	8	3	29
Veggie	2	1	1 ½	2	0	6 ½
Fruit	0	0	0	0	1	1
Fat	2	2	0	2 ½	4	10 ½

6 Meals Menu Plan

Macro	Meal 1	Meal 2	Meal 3	Meal 4	Meal 5	Meal 6	Total
Protein	5	3	6	4 ½	7 ½	3	29
Veggie	1	1	1	1 ½	2	0	6 ½
Fruit	0	0	0	0	0	1	1
Fat	2	2	1 ½	0	2	3	10 ½

Following are example menus for the weight loss formula covering normal workout and cardio days for those in the 230 pound category. You may look at the Meal Chart to pick different foods that suit your taste buds.

Example Menus

Normal Workout Days

230 lbs.

5 Meals Plan

Breakfast: ¾ cup low-fat cottage cheese mixed with 6 cherry tomatoes, 1 cup cubed cucumbers & 2 Tbs. flax seed served with 4 slices low-sodium turkey bacon; ½ cup low-sodium V-8 juice & green tea

Lunch: 8 oz. chicken breast cooked in 1 tsp. EVOO & 8 spears asparagus coated with 1 tsp. coconut oil

Post-Workout Snack: 1-⅔ scoops low-carb vanilla protein powder mixed with water & served with 1 cup sliced raw red bell pepper & 3 baby carrots

Dinner: 5 oz. lean steak & 6 oz. steamed shrimp & 1 cup steamed broccoli drizzled with 2-½ tsp. flaxseed oil

Bedtime Snack: 1 cup Greek yogurt mixed with ⅓ cup blueberries & 4 Tbs. crumbled walnuts

6 Meals Plan

Breakfast: 2 large Omega-3 eggs & 4 egg whites scrambled with 1-½ cups fresh spinach & 2 Tbs. sun-dried tomatoes, 4 slices of low-sodium turkey bacon; 1 cup green tea

Snack: 1 cup tofu cooked in 2 tsp. coconut oil & ¾ cup baked eggplant

Lunch: 9 oz. grilled red sockeye salmon on a bed of Romaine lettuce, 1 cup cucumbers & 6 cherry tomatoes drizzled wtih 1-½ tsp. flax oil

Post-Workout Snack: 1-½ scoop low-carb protein powder mixed with water & served with 1 celery stick & 9 baby carrots

Dinner: 7-½ oz. grilled flank steak, 1 cup sweet bell pepper & ½ cup chopped onions cooked in 2 tsp. EVOO

Bedtime Snack: ¾ cup low-fat cottage cheese mixed with ½ cup raspberries & 3 Tbs. pistachios

Normal Workout Blueprint

Protein: 30 blocks

Veggies: 6.5 blocks

Fruits: 1 block

Fats: 11 blocks

NORMAL WORKOUT DAYS – 240 lbs.

The weight loss formula for normal workout and cardio days includes healthy proteins, vegetables, fruits, and essential fats. We want to eliminate all starches as your body will get plenty of the right carbs through vegetables and fruits.

5 Meals Menu Plan

Macro	Meal 1	Meal 2	Meal 3	Meal 4	Meal 5	Total
Protein	5	8	5	8	4	30
Veggie	2	1	1 ½	2	0	6 ½
Fruit	0	0	0	0	1	1
Fat	2	2	0	3	4	11

6 Meals Menu Plan

Macro	Meal 1	Meal 2	Meal 3	Meal 4	Meal 5	Meal 6	Total
Protein	5	3	6	5	8	3	30
Veggie	1	1	1	1 ½	2	0	6 ½
Fruit	0	0	0	0	0	1	1
Fat	2	2	2	0	2	3	11

Following are example menus for the weight loss formula covering normal workout and cardio days for those in the 240 pound category. You may look at the Meal Chart to pick different foods that suit your taste buds.

5 Meals Plan

Breakfast: ¾ cup low-fat cottage cheese mixed with 6 cherry tomatoes, 1 cup cubed cucumbers & 2 Tbs. flax seed served with 4 slices low-sodium turkey bacon; ½ cup low-sodium V-8 juice & green tea

Lunch: 8 oz. chicken breast cooked in 1 tsp. EVOO & 8 spears asparagus coated with 1 tsp. coconut oil

Post-Workout Snack: 1-⅔ scoops low-carb vanilla protein powder mixed with water and served with 1 cup sliced raw red bell pepper & 3 baby carrots

Dinner: 5 oz. lean steak & 6 oz. steamed shrimp & 1 cup steamed broccoli drizzled with 1 Tbs. flaxseed oil

Bedtime Snack: 1-⅓ cup Greek yogurt mixed with ⅓ cup blueberries & 4 Tbs. crumbled walnuts

6 Meals Plan

Breakfast: 2 large Omega-3 eggs & 4 egg whites scrambled with 1-½ cups fresh spinach & 2 Tbs. sun-dried tomatoes, 4 slices of low-sodium turkey bacon; 1 cup green tea

Snack: 1 cup tofu cooked in 2 tsp. coconut oil & ¾ cup baked eggplant

Lunch: 9 oz. grilled red sockeye salmon on a bed of Romaine lettuce, 1 cup cucumbers & 6 cherry tomatoes drizzled wtih 2 tsp. flax oil

Post-Workout Snack: 1-⅔ scoop low-carb protein powder mixed with water & served with 1 celery stick & 9 baby carrots

Dinner: 8 oz. grilled flank steak, 1 cup sweet bell pepper & ½ cup chopped onions cooked in 2 tsp. EVOO

Bedtime Snack: ¾ cup low-fat cottage cheese mixed with ½ cup raspberries & 3 Tbs. pistachios

Normal Workout Blueprint

Protein: 31 blocks

Veggies: 7 blocks

Fruits: 1 block

Fats: 11.5 blocks

NORMAL WORKOUT DAYS – 250 lbs.

The weight loss formula for normal workout and cardio days includes healthy proteins, vegetables, fruits, and essential fats. We want to eliminate all starches as your body will get plenty of the right carbs through vegetables and fruits.

5 Meals Menu Plan

Macro	Meal 1	Meal 2	Meal 3	Meal 4	Meal 5	Total
Protein	5	8	6	8	4	31
Veggie	2	1	2	2	0	7
Fruit	0	0	0	0	1	1
Fat	2	2 ½	0	3	4	11 ½

6 Meals Menu Plan

Macro	Meal 1	Meal 2	Meal 3	Meal 4	Meal 5	Meal 6	Total
Protein	5	3	6	5	8	4	31
Veggie	1	1	1	2	2	0	7
Fruit	0	0	0	0	0	1	1
Fat	2	2	2	0	2	3 ½	11 ½

Following are example menus for the weight loss formula covering normal workout and cardio days for those in the 250 pound category. You may look at the Meal Chart to pick different foods that suit your taste buds.

Example Menus

Normal Workout Days

250 lbs.

5 Meals Plan

Breakfast: ¾ cup low-fat cottage cheese mixed with 6 cherry tomatoes, 1 cup cubed cucumbers & 2 Tbs. flax seed served with 4 slices low-sodium turkey bacon; ½ cup low-sodium V-8 juice & green tea

Lunch: 8 oz. chicken breast cooked in 1-½ tsp. EVOO & 8 spears asparagus coated with 1 tsp. coconut oil

Post-Workout Snack: 2 scoops low-carb vanilla protein powder mixed with water and served with 1 cup sliced raw red bell pepper & 6 baby carrots

Dinner: 5 oz. lean steak & 6 oz. steamed shrimp & 1 cup steamed broccoli drizzled with 1 Tbs. flaxseed oil

Bedtime Snack: 1-⅓ cup Greek yogurt mixed with ⅓ cup blueberries & 4 Tbs. crumbled walnuts

6 Meals Plan

Breakfast: 2 large Omega-3 eggs & 4 egg whites scrambled with 1-½ cups fresh spinach & 2 Tbs. sun-dried tomatoes, 4 slices of low-sodium turkey bacon; 1 cup green tea

Snack: 1 cup tofu cooked in 2 tsp. coconut oil & ¾ cup baked eggplant

Lunch: 9 oz. grilled red sockeye salmon on a bed of Romaine lettuce, 1 cup cucumbers & 6 cherry tomatoes drizzled wtih 2 tsp. flax oil

Post-Workout Snack: 1-⅔ scoop low-carb protein powder mixed with water & served with 1 cup sliced cucumbers, 6 baby carrots & 1 cup raw red bell pepper slices

Dinner: 8 oz. grilled flank steak, 1 cup sweet bell pepper & ½ cup chopped onions cooked in 2 tsp. EVOO

Bedtime Snack: 1-⅓ cup low-fat cottage cheese mixed with ½ cup raspberries & 3-½ Tbs. pistachios

Normal Workout Blueprint	NORMAL WORKOUT DAYS – 260 lbs.

Normal Workout Blueprint

Protein: 32.5 blocks

Veggies: 7.5 blocks

Fruits: 1 block

Fats: 12 blocks

NORMAL WORKOUT DAYS – 260 lbs.

The weight loss formula for normal workout and cardio days includes healthy proteins, vegetables, fruits, and essential fats. We want to eliminate all starches as your body will get plenty of the right carbs through vegetables and fruits.

5 Meals Menu Plan

Macro	Meal 1	Meal 2	Meal 3	Meal 4	Meal 5	Total
Protein	5	8	6	8	5 ½	32 ½
Veggie	2	1 ½	2	2	0	7 ½
Fruit	0	0	0	0	1	1
Fat	2	3	0	3	4	12

6 Meals Menu Plan

Macro	Meal 1	Meal 2	Meal 3	Meal 4	Meal 5	Meal 6	Total
Protein	5	3	6	6	8	4 ½	32 ½
Veggie	1 ½	1	1	2	2	0	7 ½
Fruit	0	0	0	0	0	1	1
Fat	2	2	2	0	2	4	12

Following are example menus for the weight loss formula covering normal workout and cardio days for those in the 260 pound category. You may look at the Meal Chart to pick different foods that suit your taste buds.

5 Meals Plan

Breakfast: ¾ cup low-fat cottage cheese mixed with 6 cherry tomatoes, 1 cup cubed cucumbers & 2 Tbs. flax seed served with 4 slices low-sodium turkey bacon; ½ cup low-sodium V-8 juice & green tea

Lunch: 8 oz. chicken breast cooked in 2 tsp. EVOO & 12 spears asparagus coated with 1 tsp. coconut oil

Post-Workout Snack: 2 scoops low-carb vanilla protein powder mixed with water & served with 1 cup sliced raw red bell pepper & 6 baby carrots

Dinner: 5 oz. lean steak & 6 oz. steamed shrimp & 1 cup steamed broccoli drizzled with 1 Tbs. flaxseed oil

Bedtime Snack: 1 cup Greek yogurt mixed with ⅓ cup blueberries & 4 Tbs. crumbled walnuts ; ¾ scoop chocolate protein powder mixed with water

6 Meals Plan

Breakfast: 2 large Omega-3 eggs & 4 egg whites scrambled with 1-½ cups fresh spinach & 2 Tbs. sun-dried tomatoes, 4 slices of low-sodium turkey bacon; 1 cup green tea

Snack: 1 cup tofu cooked in 2 tsp. coconut oil & ¾ cup baked eggplant

Lunch: 9 oz. grilled red sockeye salmon on a bed of Romaine lettuce, 1 cup cucumbers & 6 cherry tomatoes drizzled wtih 2 tsp. flax oil

Post-Workout Snack: 2 scoops low-carb protein powder mixed with water & served with 1 cup sliced cucumbers, 6 baby carrots & 1 cup raw red bell pepper slices

Bedtime Snack: 1 cup low-fat cottage cheese mixed with ½ scoop chocolate protein powder, ½ cup raspberries, 4 Tbs. pistachios & a little water

Normal Workout Blueprint

Protein: 34 blocks

Veggies: 7.5 blocks

Fruits: 1 block

Fats: 12.5 blocks

NORMAL WORKOUT DAYS – 270 lbs.

The weight loss formula for normal workout and cardio days includes healthy proteins, vegetables, fruits, and essential fats. We want to eliminate all starches as your body will get plenty of the right carbs through vegetables and fruits.

5 Meals Menu Plan

Macro	Meal 1	Meal 2	Meal 3	Meal 4	Meal 5	Total
Protein	5	8	6	8	7	34
Veggie	2	1 ½	2	2	0	7 ½
Fruit	0	0	0	0	1	1
Fat	2 ½	3	0	3	4	12 ½

6 Meals Menu Plan

Macro	Meal 1	Meal 2	Meal 3	Meal 4	Meal 5	Meal 6	Total
Protein	5	3	6	6	8	6	34
Veggie	1 ½	1	1	2	2	0	7 ½
Fruit	0	0	0	0	0	1	1
Fat	2	2	2	0	2 ½	4	12 ½

Following are example menus for the weight loss formula covering normal workout and cardio days for those in the 270 pound category. You may look at the Meal Chart to pick different foods that suit your taste buds.

5 Meals Plan

Breakfast: ¾ cup low-fat cottage cheese mixed with 6 cherry tomatoes, 1 cup cubed cucumbers & 2-½ Tbs. flax seed served with 4 slices low-sodium turkey bacon; ½ cup low-sodium V-8 juice & green tea

Lunch: 8 oz. chicken breast cooked in 2 tsp. EVOO & 12 spears asparagus coated with 1 tsp. coconut oil

Post-Workout Snack: 2 scoops low-carb vanilla protein powder mixed with water & served with 1 cup sliced raw red bell pepper & 6 baby carrots

Dinner: 5 oz. lean steak & 6 oz. steamed shrimp & 1 cup steamed broccoli drizzled with 1 Tbs. flaxseed oil

Bedtime Snack: 1 cup Greek yogurt mixed with ⅓ cup blueberries & 4 Tbs. crumbled walnuts ; 1-⅓ scoops chocolate protein powder mixed with water

6 Meals Plan

Breakfast: 2 large Omega-3 eggs & 4 egg whites scrambled with 1-½ cups fresh spinach & 2 Tbs. sun-dried tomatoes, 4 slices of low-sodium turkey bacon; 1 cup green tea

Snack: 1 cup tofu cooked in 2 tsp. coconut oil & ¾ cup baked eggplant

Lunch: 9 oz. grilled red sockeye salmon on a bed of Romaine lettuce, 1 cup cucumbers & 6 cherry tomatoes drizzled wtih 2 tsp. flax oil

Post-Workout Snack: 2 scoops low-carb protein powder mixed with water & served with 1 cup sliced cucumbers , 6 baby carrots & 1 cup raw red bell pepper slices

Dinner: 8 oz. grilled flank steak, 1 cup sweet bell pepper & ½ cup chopped onions cooked in 2-½ tsp. EVOO

Bedtime Snack: 1 cup low-fat cottage cheese mixed with ⅔ scoop chocolate protein powder , ½ cup raspberries & 4 Tbs. pistachios & a little water

NORMAL WORKOUT DAYS – 280 lbs.

The weight loss formula for normal workout and cardio days includes healthy proteins, vegetables, fruits, and essential fats. We want to eliminate all starches as your body will get plenty of the right carbs through vegetables and fruits.

5 Meals Menu Plan

Macro	Meal 1	Meal 2	Meal 3	Meal 4	Meal 5	Total
Protein	6	8	6	8	7	35
Veggie	2	2	2	2	0	8
Fruit	0	0	0	0	1	1
Fat	3	3	0	3	4	13

6 Meals Menu Plan

Macro	Meal 1	Meal 2	Meal 3	Meal 4	Meal 5	Meal 6	Total
Protein	5	4	6	6	8	6	35
Veggie	2	1	1	2	2	0	8
Fruit	0	0	0	0	0	1	1
Fat	2	2	3	0	2	4	13

Following are example menus for the weight loss formula covering normal workout and cardio days for those in the 280 pound category. You may look at the Meal Chart to pick different foods that suit your taste buds.

5 Meals Plan

Breakfast: 1 cup low-fat cottage cheese mixed with 6 cherry tomatoes, 1 cup cubed cucumbers & 3 Tbs. flax seed served with 4 slices low-sodium turkey bacon; ½ cup low-sodium V-8 juice & green tea

Lunch: 8 oz. chicken breast cooked in 2 tsp. EVOO & 8 spears asparagus & 6 baby carrots coated with 1 tsp. coconut oil

Post-Workout Snack: 2 scoops low-carb vanilla protein powder mixed with water & served with 1 cup sliced raw red bell pepper & 6 baby carrots

Dinner: 5 oz. lean steak & 6 oz. steamed shrimp & 1 cup steamed broccoli drizzled with 1 Tbs. flaxseed oil

Bedtime Snack: 1 cup Greek yogurt mixed with ⅓ cup blueberries & 4 Tbs. crumbled walnuts ; 1-⅓ scoops chocolate protein powder mixed with water

6 Meals Plan

Breakfast: 2 large Omega-3 eggs & 4 egg whites scrambled with 1-½ cups fresh spinach & 2 Tbs. sun-dried tomatoes, 4 slices of low-sodium turkey bacon; 1 cup green tea

Snack: 1-⅓ cup tofu cooked in 2 tsp. coconut oil & ¾ cup baked eggplant

Lunch: 9 oz. grilled red sockeye salmon on a bed of Romaine lettuce, 1 cup cucumbers & 6 cherry tomatoes drizzled wtih 1 TBS. flax oil

Post-Workout Snack: 2 scoops low-carb protein powder mixed with water & served with 1 cup sliced cucumbers, 6 baby carrots & 1 cup raw red pepper slices

Dinner: 8 oz. grilled flank steak, 1 cup sweet bell pepper & ½ cup chopped onions cooked in 2 tsp. EVOO

Bedtime Snack: 1 cup low-fat cottage cheese mixed with ⅔ scoop chocolate protein powder , ½ cup raspberries, 4 Tbs. pistachios & a little water

10 – Blueprints & Examples for Strenuous Weight Training Days

What are strenuous training days?

✓ Strenuous weight training includes any workouts that force your muscles to resist some form of weight, as well as exert the most energy of all the days.

✓ Strenuous weight training may include the use of exercise equipment (i.e., dumbbells, barbells, or weight machines). It may even include the use of your own body weight for resistance such as with plyometric or crossfit training.

✓ On an intensity scale of 1 to 10, where 1 equates to no effort and 10 equate to all-out effort, a strenuous intensity level would be 8 to 10.

When to Use this Blueprint

Use this blueprint for one or two of your most strenuous weight or resistance training days per week. This blueprint is also for those who have laborious jobs. For fastest results on body fat loss, do not use this formula for more than two days per week.

What Foods this Blueprint Includes

This blueprint will provide more calories to supply your body with the extra energy it will need on strenuous workout days, yet only enough to still allow you to burn body fat. Proteins are included to nourish your body, keep you satiated, preserve lean muscle mass, and keep your metabolism on fire. Vegetable carbohydrates are built in to supply your body with vitamins, minerals, and phytonutrients. Vegetables will also protect your body from damaging free radicals by providing it with antioxidants. The fiber in vegetables will help rid your body of metabolic waste. A small portion of fruit carbohydrates are included to replenish your muscles and brain with energy. Just enough lentil, whole grain, and tuber carbohydrates are added to replenish your body with nutrient and energy that was depleted from the strenuous workouts, as well as the normal and cardio workouts from the week. By including these healthy starchy carbohydrates once or twice per week, your metabolism will be recharged. Dietary fats will balance out your meals and will help supply you with essential nutrients for every cell in your body to function optimally. You should exclude fats in your post-workout meal.

How to Count Blocks of Food

An example of counting blocks of food has been given in Chapter 7. However, a new example detailing this particular blueprint has been given below.

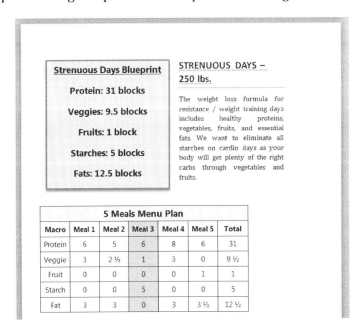

For this component of Phase 3 nutrition planning, you have the option of choosing from five or six meals per day. The example just given shows the "5 Meals Menu Plan." At the top of each page, you will see the blocks of food allotted for this weight category. There are 31 protein blocks, 9.5 vegetable blocks, 1 fruit block, 5 starch blocks, and 12.5 fat blocks for the "5 Meals Menu Plan" of the 250 pound menu plan. The meal shaded in gray (Meal 3) is your post workout meal which includes your starchy carbohydrates yet excludes your dietary fat. On the opposite page, you will be given examples for each menu plan as shown below.

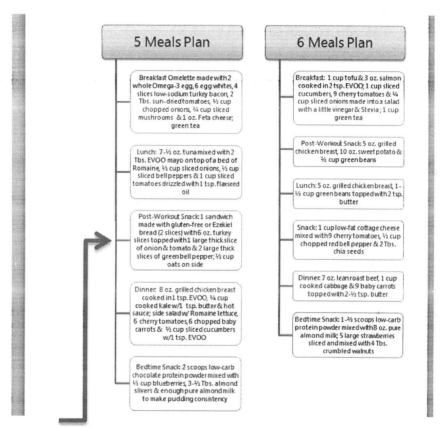

On the 250 pound menu plan, you will see how many blocks are allotted for each meal. Look at Meal 3. It includes 6 protein blocks, 1 veggie block, 0 fruit blocks, 5 starch blocks, and 0 fat blocks. If you then look at the snack meal example for the "5 Meals Menu Plan" above, you will see that that it consists of 6 ounces of turkey (6 proteins), 2 large slices of green bell pepper (1 veggie), as well as two slices of Ezekiel bread and ¾ cup oats (5 starches). The foods selected are taken from the meal charts in Chapter 12 to find the serving size of each food by using the block number given on the menu plan multiplied by the serving size given on the meal charts. You may refer to Chapter 7 to determine correct calculations.

Strenuous Days Blueprint

Protein: 15 blocks

Veggies: 4 blocks

Fruits: 1 block

Starches: 2.5 blocks

Fats: 6 blocks

STRENUOUS DAYS – 120 lbs.

The weight loss formula for resistance/weight training days includes healthy proteins, vegetables, fruits, and essential fats. We will also add starches as your body will need to replenish glycogen and recharge your metabolism. This blueprint should be used 1-2 times per week.

5 Meals Menu Plan

Macro	Meal 1	Meal 2	Meal 3	Meal 4	Meal 5	Total
Protein	3	3	3	3	3	15
Veggie	1	1	1	1	0	4
Fruit	0	0	0	0	1	1
Starch	0	0	2 ½	0	0	2 ½
Fat	2	1	0	2	1	6

6 Meals Menu Plan

Macro	Meal 1	Meal 2	Meal 3	Meal 4	Meal 5	Meal 6	Total
Protein	3	2	3	2	3	2	15
Veggie	1	½	1	½	1	0	4
Fruit	0	0	0	0	0	1	1
Starch	0	2 ½	0	0	0	0	2 ½
Fat	2	0	1	1	1	1	6

Following are example menus for the weight loss formula covering resistance/weight training days for those in the 120 pound category. You may look at the Meal Chart to pick different foods that suit your taste buds.

Example Menus

Strenuous Days

120 lbs.

5 Meals Plan

Breakfast Omelette made with 1 whole Omega-3 egg, 3 egg whites, 2 slices low-sodium turkey bacon, 2 Tbs. sun-dried tomatoes & 1 oz. Feta cheese; green tea

Lunch: 4.5 oz. tuna mixed with 1 Tbs. EVOO mayo on top of a bed of Romaine, 1 cup sliced cucumbers & 1 cup sliced tomatoes

Post-Workout Snack: ½ sandwich made with gluten-free or Ezekiel bread (1 slice) with 3 oz. turkey slices topped with 1 large thick slice of onion & tomato & 2 large thick slices of green bell pepper; ¼ cup oats on side

Dinner: 3 oz. grilled chicken breast cooked in 1 tsp. EVOO, ¾ cup cooked kale with 1 tsp. butter & hot sauce

Bedtime Snack: 1 scoop low-carb chocolate protein powder mixed with ⅓ cup blueberries, 1 Tbs. almond slivers & enough pure almond milk to make pudding consistency

6 Meals Plan

Breakfast: 1 cup tofu cooked in 2 tsp. EVOO; 1 cup sliced cucumbers, ½ cup sliced tomatoes & ¼ cup sliced onions made into a salad with a little vinegar & Stevia ; 1 cup green tea

Post-Workout Snack: 2 oz. grilled chicken breast, 5 oz. sweet potato & ⅓ cup green beans

Lunch: 3 oz. grilled chicken breast, ⅔ cup green beans topped with 1 tsp. butter

Snack: ½ cup low-fat cottage cheese mixed with 3 cherry tomatoes & 1 Tbs. chia seeds

Dinner: 3 oz. lean roast beef, 1 cup cooked cabbage topped with 1 tsp. butter

Bedtime Snack: ⅔ scoop low-carb protein powder mixed with 8 oz. pure almond milk; 5 large strawberries sliced and mixed with 1 Tbs. crumbled walnuts

Strenuous Days Blueprint

Protein: 16 blocks

Veggies: 4.5 blocks

Fruits: 1 block

Starches: 2.5 blocks

Fats: 6.5 blocks

STRENUOUS DAYS – 130 lbs.

The weight loss formula for resistance/weight training days includes healthy proteins, vegetables, fruits, and essential fats. We will also add starches as your body will need to replenish glycogen and recharge your metabolism. This blueprint should be used 1-2 times per week.

5 Meals Menu Plan

Macro	Meal 1	Meal 2	Meal 3	Meal 4	Meal 5	Total
Protein	3	3	3	4	3	16
Veggie	1	1	1	1 ½	0	4 ½
Fruit	0	0	0	0	1	1
Starch	0	0	2 ½	0	0	2 ½
Fat	2	1	0	2	1 ½	6 ½

6 Meals Menu Plan

Macro	Meal 1	Meal 2	Meal 3	Meal 4	Meal 5	Meal 6	Total
Protein	3	2	3	2	3	3	16
Veggie	1	½	1	1	1	0	4 ½
Fruit	0	0	0	0	0	1	1
Starch	0	2 ½	0	0	0	0	2 ½
Fat	2	0	1	1	1	1 ½	6 ½

Following are example menus for the weight loss formula covering resistance/weight training days for those in the 130 pound category. You may look at the Meal Chart to pick different foods that suit your taste buds.

Example Menus

Strenuous Days

130 lbs.

5 Meals Plan

Breakfast Omelette made with 1 whole Omega-3 egg, 3 egg whites, 2 slices low-sodium turkey bacon, 2 Tbs. sun-dried tomatoes & 1 oz. Feta cheese; green tea

Lunch: 4.5 oz. tuna mixed with 1 Tbs. EVOO mayo on top of a bed of Romaine, 1 cup sliced cucumbers & 1 cup sliced tomatoes

Post-Workout Snack: ½ sandwich made with gluten-free or Ezekiel bread (1 slice) with 3 oz. turkey slices topped with 1 large thick slice of onion & tomato & 2 large thick slices of green bell pepper; ¼ cup oats on side

Dinner: 4 oz. grilled chicken breast cooked in 1 tsp. EVOO, 1 heaping cup cooked kale with 1 tsp. butter & hot sauce

Bedtime Snack: 1 scoop low-carb chocolate protein powder mixed with ⅓ cup blueberries, 1-½ Tbs. almond slivers & enough pure almond milk to make pudding consistency

6 Meals Plan

Breakfast: 1 cup tofu cooked in 2 tsp. EVOO; 1 cup sliced cucumbers, ½ cup sliced tomatoes & ¼ cup sliced onions made into a salad with a little vinegar & Stevia ; 1 cup green tea

Post-Workout Snack: 2 oz. grilled chicken breast, 5 oz. sweet potato & ⅓ cup green beans

Lunch: 3 oz. grilled chicken breast, ⅔ cup green beans topped with 1 tsp. butter

Snack: ½ cup low-fat cottage cheese mixed with 6 cherry tomatoes & 1 Tbs. chia seeds

Dinner: 3 oz. lean roast beef, 1 cup cooked cabbage topped with 1 tsp. butter

Bedtime Snack: 1 scoop low-carb protein powder mixed with 8 oz. pure almond milk; 5 large strawberries sliced and mixed with 1-½ Tbs. crumbled walnuts

Strenuous Days Blueprint

Protein: 17.5 blocks

Veggies: 5 blocks

Fruits: 1 block

Starches: 3 blocks

Fats: 7 blocks

STRENUOUS DAYS – 140 lbs.

The weight loss formula for resistance/weight training days includes healthy proteins, vegetables, fruits, and essential fats. We will also add starches as your body will need to replenish glycogen and recharge your metabolism. This blueprint should be used 1-2 times per week.

5 Meals Menu Plan

Macro	Meal 1	Meal 2	Meal 3	Meal 4	Meal 5	Total
Protein	3 ½	3	4	4	3	17 ½
Veggie	2	1	1	1	0	5
Fruit	0	0	0	0	1	1
Starch	0	0	3	0	0	3
Fat	2	1	0	2	2	7

6 Meals Menu Plan

Macro	Meal 1	Meal 2	Meal 3	Meal 4	Meal 5	Meal 6	Total
Protein	3	3	3	2 ½	3	3	17 ½
Veggie	1	1	1	1	1	0	5
Fruit	0	0	0	0	0	1	1
Starch	0	3	0	0	0	0	3
Fat	2	0	1	1	1	2	7

Following are example menus for the weight loss formula covering resistance/weight training days for those in the 140 pound category. You may look at the Meal Chart to pick different foods that suit your taste buds.

Example Menus

Strenuous Days

140 lbs.

5 Meals Plan

Breakfast Omelette made with 1 whole Omega-3 egg, 4 egg whites, 2 slices low-sodium turkey bacon, 2 Tbs. sun-dried tomatoes, ½ cup chopped onions & 1 oz. Feta cheese; green tea

Lunch: 4.5 oz. tuna mixed with 1 Tbs. EVOO mayo on top of a bed of Romaine, 1 cup sliced cucumbers & 1 cup sliced tomatoes

Post-Workout Snack: ½ sandwich made with gluten-free or Ezekiel bread (1 slice) with 4 oz. turkey slices topped with 1 large thick slice of onion & tomato & 2 large thick slices of green bell pepper; ½ cup oats on side

Dinner: 4 oz. grilled chicken breast cooked in 1 tsp. EVOO, ¾ cup cooked kale with 1 tsp. butter & hot sauce

Bedtime Snack: 1 scoop low-carb chocolate protein powder mixed with ⅓ cup blueberries, 2 Tbs. almond slivers & enough pure almond milk to make pudding consistency

6 Meals Plan

Breakfast: 1 cup tofu cooked in 2 tsp. EVOO; 1 cup sliced cucumbers, ½ cup sliced tomatoes & ¼ cup sliced onions made into a salad with a little vinegar & Stevia ; 1 cup green tea

Post-Workout Snack: 3 oz. grilled chicken breast, 6 oz. sweet potato & ⅔ cup green beans

Lunch: 3 oz. grilled chicken breast, ⅔ cup green beans topped with 1 tsp. butter

Snack: ⅔ cup low-fat cottage cheese mixed with 6 cherry tomatoes & 1 Tbs. chia seeds

Dinner: 3 oz. lean roast beef, 1 cup cooked cabbage topped with 1 tsp. butter

Bedtime Snack: 1 scoop low-carb protein powder mixed with 8 oz. pure almond milk; 5 large strawberries sliced and mixed with 2 Tbs. crumbled walnuts

Strenuous Days Blueprint

Protein: 19 blocks

Veggies: 5 blocks

Fruits: 1 block

Starches: 3 blocks

Fats: 7.5 blocks

STRENUOUS DAYS – 150 lbs.

The weight loss formula for resistance/weight training days includes healthy proteins, vegetables, fruits, and essential fats. We will also add starches as your body will need to replenish glycogen and recharge your metabolism. This blueprint should be used 1-2 times per week.

5 Meals Menu Plan

Macro	Meal 1	Meal 2	Meal 3	Meal 4	Meal 5	Total
Protein	4	3	4	5	3	19
Veggie	2	1	1	1	0	5
Fruit	0	0	0	0	1	1
Starch	0	0	3	0	0	3
Fat	2	1	0	2	2 ½	7 ½

6 Meals Menu Plan

Macro	Meal 1	Meal 2	Meal 3	Meal 4	Meal 5	Meal 6	Total
Protein	3	3	3	3	4	3	19
Veggie	1	1	1	1	1	0	5
Fruit	0	0	0	0	0	1	1
Starch	0	3	0	0	0	0	3
Fat	2	0	1	1	1	2 ½	7 ½

Following are example menus for the weight loss formula covering resistance/weight training days for those in the 150 pound category. You may look at the Meal Chart to pick different foods that suit your taste buds.

Example Menus

Strenuous Days

150 lbs.

5 Meals Plan

Breakfast Omelette made with 1 whole Omega-3 egg, 5 egg whites, 2 slices low-sodium turkey bacon, 2 Tbs. sun-dried tomatoes, ½ cup chopped onions & 1 oz. Feta cheese; green tea

Lunch: 4.5 oz. tuna mixed with 1 Tbs. EVOO mayo on top of a bed of Romaine, 1 cup sliced cucumbers & 1 cup sliced tomatoes

Post-Workout Snack: ½ sandwich made with gluten-free or Ezekiel bread (1 slice) with 4 oz. turkey slices topped with 1 large thick slice of onion & tomato & 2 large thick slices of green bell pepper; ½ cup oats on side

Dinner: 5 oz. grilled chicken breast cooked in 1 tsp. EVOO, ¾ cup cooked kale with 1 tsp. butter & hot sauce

Bedtime Snack: 1 scoop low-carb chocolate protein powder mixed with ⅓ cup blueberries, 2-½ Tbs. almond slivers & enough pure almond milk to make pudding consistency

6 Meals Plan

Breakfast: 1 cup tofu cooked in 2 tsp. EVOO; 1 cup sliced cucumbers, ½ cup sliced tomatoes & ¼ cup sliced onions made into a salad with a little vinegar & Stevia ; 1 cup green tea

Post- Workout Snack: 3 oz. grilled chicken breast, 6 oz. sweet potato & ⅔ cup green beans

Lunch: 3 oz. grilled chicken breast, ⅔ cup green beans topped with 1 tsp. butter

Snack: ¾ cup low-fat cottage cheese mixed with 6 cherry tomatoes & 1 Tbs. chia seeds

Dinner: 4 oz. lean roast beef, 1 cup cooked cabbage topped with 1 tsp. butter

Bedtime Snack: 1 scoop low-carb protein powder mixed with 8 oz. pure almond milk; 5 large strawberries sliced and mixed with 2-½ Tbs. crumbled walnuts

Strenuous Days Blueprint

Protein: 20 blocks

Veggies: 5.5 blocks

Fruits: 1 block

Starches: 3.5 blocks

Fats: 8 blocks

STRENUOUS DAYS – 160 lbs.

The weight loss formula for resistance/weight training days includes healthy proteins, vegetables, fruits, and essential fats. We will also add starches as your body will need to replenish glycogen and recharge your metabolism. This blueprint should be used 1-2 times per week.

5 Meals Menu Plan

Macro	Meal 1	Meal 2	Meal 3	Meal 4	Meal 5	Total
Protein	4	4	4	5	3	20
Veggie	2	1	1	1 ½	0	5 ½
Fruit	0	0	0	0	1	1
Starch	0	0	3 ½	0	0	3 ½
Fat	2	1	0	2	3	8

6 Meals Menu Plan

Macro	Meal 1	Meal 2	Meal 3	Meal 4	Meal 5	Meal 6	Total
Protein	3	3	4	3	4	3	20
Veggie	1	1	1	1	1 ½	0	5 ½
Fruit	0	0	0	0	0	1	1
Starch	0	3 ½	0	0	0	0	3 ½
Fat	2	0	1	1	1	3	8

Following are example menus for the weight loss formula covering resistance/weight training days for those in the 160 pound category. You may look at the Meal Chart to pick different foods that suit your taste buds.

5 Meals Plan

Breakfast Omelette made with 1 whole Omega-3 egg, 5 egg whites, 2 slices low-sodium turkey bacon, 2 Tbs. sun-dried tomatoes, ½ cup chopped onions & 1 oz. Feta cheese; green tea

Lunch: 6 oz. tuna mixed with 1 Tbs. EVOO mayo on top of a bed of Romaine, 1 cup sliced cucumbers & 1 cup sliced tomatoes

Post-Workout Snack: ½ sandwich made with gluten-free or Ezekiel bread (1 slice) with 4 oz. turkey slices topped with 1 large thick slice of onion & tomato & 2 large thick slices of green bell pepper; ¾ cup oats on side

Dinner: 5 oz. grilled chicken breast cooked in 1 tsp. EVOO, 1 heaping cup cooked kale with 1 tsp. butter & hot sauce

Bedtime Snack: 1 scoop low-carb chocolate protein powder mixed with ⅓ cup blueberries, 3 Tbs. almond slivers & enough pure almond milk to make pudding consistency

6 Meals Plan

Breakfast: 1 cup tofu cooked in 2 tsp. EVOO; 1 cup sliced cucumbers, ½ cup slied tomatoes & ¼ cup sliced onions made into a salad with a little vinegar & Stevia ; 1 cup green tea

Post-Workout Snack: 3 oz. grilled chicken breast, 7 oz. sweet potato & ⅔ cup green beans

Lunch: 4 oz. grilled chicken breast, ⅔ cup green beans topped with 1 tsp. butter

Snack: ¾ cup low-fat cottage cheese mixed with 6 cherry tomatoes & 1 Tbs. chia seeds

Dinner: 4 oz. lean roast beef, 1-½ cups cooked cabbage topped with 1 tsp. butter

Bedtime Snack: 1 scoop low-carb protein powder mixed with 8 oz. pure almond milk; 5 large strawberries sliced and mixed with 3 Tbs. crumbled walnuts

Strenuous Days Blueprint

Protein: 21 blocks

Veggies: 6 blocks

Fruits: 1 block

Starches: 3.5 blocks

Fats: 8.5 blocks

STRENUOUS DAYS – 170 lbs.

The weight loss formula for resistance/weight training days includes healthy proteins, vegetables, fruits, and essential fats. We will also add starches as your body will need to replenish glycogen and recharge your metabolism. This blueprint should be used 1-2 times per week.

5 Meals Menu Plan

Macro	Meal 1	Meal 2	Meal 3	Meal 4	Meal 5	Total
Protein	5	4	4	5	3	21
Veggie	2	1	1	2	0	6
Fruit	0	0	0	0	1	1
Starch	0	0	3 ½	0	0	3 ½
Fat	2	1 ½	0	2	3	8 ½

6 Meals Menu Plan

Macro	Meal 1	Meal 2	Meal 3	Meal 4	Meal 5	Meal 6	Total
Protein	4	3	4	3	4	3	21
Veggie	1	1	1	1	2	0	6
Fruit	0	0	0	0	0	1	1
Starch	0	3 ½	0	0	0	0	3 ½
Fat	2	0	1	1	1 ½	3	8 ½

Following are example menus for the weight loss formula covering resistance/weight training days for those in the 170 pound category. You may look at the Meal Chart to pick different foods that suit your taste buds.

5 Meals Plan

Breakfast Omelette made with 1 whole Omega-3 egg, 5 egg whites, 4 slices low-sodium turkey bacon, 4 Tbs. sun-dried tomatoes, ½ cup chopped onions & 1 oz. Feta cheese; green tea

Lunch: 6 oz. tuna mixed with 1-½ Tbs. EVOO mayo on top of a bed of Romaine, 1 cup sliced cucumbers & 1 cup sliced tomatoes

Post-Workout Snack: ½ sandwich made with gluten-free or Ezekiel bread (1 slice) with 4 oz. turkey slices topped with 1 large thick slice of onion & tomato & 2 large thick slices of green bell pepper; ¾ cup oats on side

Dinner: 5 oz. grilled chicken breast cooked in 1 tsp. EVOO, 1-½ cups cooked kale with 1 tsp. butter & hot sauce

Bedtime Snack: 1 scoop low-carb chocolate protein powder mixed with ⅓ cup blueberries, 3 Tbs. almond slivers & enough pure almond milk to make pudding consistency

6 Meals Plan

Breakfast: 1-⅓ cup tofu cooked in 2 tsp. EVOO; 1 cup sliced cucumbers , ½ cup sliced tomatoes & ¼ cup sliced onions made into a salad with a little vinegar & Stevia ; 1 cup green tea

Post-Workout Snack: 3 oz. grilled chicken breast, 7 oz. sweet potato & ⅔ cup green beans

Lunch: 4 oz. grilled chicken breast, ⅔ cup green beans topped with 1 tsp. butter

Snack: ¾ cup low-fat cottage cheese mixed with 6 cherry tomatoes & 1 Tbs. chia seeds

Dinner: 4 oz. lean roast beef, 1 cup cooked cabbage & 6 baby carrots topped with 1-½ tsp. butter

Bedtime Snack: 1 scoop low-carb protein powder mixed with 8 oz. pure almond milk; 5 large strawberries sliced and mixed with 3 Tbs. crumbled walnuts

Strenuous Days Blueprint

Protein: 22.5 blocks

Veggies: 6.5 blocks

Fruits: 1 block

Starches: 4 blocks

Fats: 9 blocks

STRENUOUS DAYS – 180 lbs.

The weight loss formula for resistance/weight training days includes healthy proteins, vegetables, fruits, and essential fats. We will also add starches as your body will need to replenish glycogen and recharge your metabolism. This blueprint should be used 1-2 times per week.

5 Meals Menu Plan

Macro	Meal 1	Meal 2	Meal 3	Meal 4	Meal 5	Total
Protein	5	4	4	5 ½	4	22 ½
Veggie	2 ½	1	1	2	0	6 ½
Fruit	0	0	0	0	1	1
Starch	0	0	4	0	0	4
Fat	2	2	0	2	3	9

6 Meals Menu Plan

Macro	Meal 1	Meal 2	Meal 3	Meal 4	Meal 5	Meal 6	Total
Protein	4	3	4	3 ½	5	3	22 ½
Veggie	1	1	1 ½	1	2	0	6 ½
Fruit	0	0	0	0	0	1	1
Starch	0	4	0	0	0	0	4
Fat	2	0	1	1	2	3	9

Following are example menus for the weight loss formula covering resistance/weight training days for those in the 180 pound category. You may look at the Meal Chart to pick different foods that suit your taste buds.

Example Menus

Strenuous Days

180 lbs.

5 Meals Plan

Breakfast Omelette made with 1 whole Omega-3 egg, 5 egg whites, 4 slices low-sodium turkey bacon, 4-½ Tbs. sun-dried tomatoes, ½ cup chopped onions & 1 oz. Feta cheese; green tea

Lunch: 6 oz. tuna mixed with 2 Tbs. EVOO mayo on top of a bed of Romaine, 1 cup sliced cucumbers & 1 cup sliced tomatoes

Post-Workout Snack: 1 sandwich made with gluten-free or Ezekiel bread (2 slices) with 4 oz. turkey slices topped with 1 large thick slice of onion & tomato & 2 large thick slices of green bell pepper

Dinner: 5-½ oz. grilled chicken breast cooked in 1 tsp. EVOO, 1-½ cups cooked kale with 1 tsp. butter & hot sauce

Bedtime Snack: 1-⅓ scoop low-carb chocolate protein powder mixed with ⅓ cup blueberries, 3 Tbs. almond slivers & enough pure almond milk to make pudding consistency

6 Meals Plan

Breakfast: 1-⅓ cup tofu cooked in 2 tsp. EVOO; 1 cup sliced cucumbers, ½ cup sliced tomatoes & ¼ cup sliced onions made into a salad with a little vinegar & Stevia ; 1 cup green tea

Post-Workout Snack: 3 oz. grilled chicken breast, 8 oz. sweet potato, ⅔ cup green beans

Lunch: 4 oz. grilled chicken breast, 1 cup green beans topped with 1 tsp. butter

Snack: ¾ heaping cup low-fat cottage cheese mixed with 6 cherry tomatoes & 1 Tbs. chia seeds

Dinner: 5 oz. lean roast beef, 1 cup cooked cabbage & 6 baby carrots topped with 2 tsp. butter

Bedtime Snack: 1 scoop low-carb protein powder mixed with 8 oz. pure almond milk; 5 large strawberries sliced and mixed with 3 Tbs. crumbled walnuts

Strenuous Days Blueprint

Protein: 24 blocks

Veggies: 7 blocks

Fruits: 1 block

Starches: 4 blocks

Fats: 9.5 blocks

STRENUOUS DAYS – 190 lbs.

The weight loss formula for resistance/weight training days includes healthy proteins, vegetables, fruits, and essential fats. We will also add starches as your body will need to replenish glycogen and recharge your metabolism. This blueprint should be used 1-2 times per week.

5 Meals Menu Plan

Macro	Meal 1	Meal 2	Meal 3	Meal 4	Meal 5	Total
Protein	5	4	4 ½	6 ½	4	24
Veggie	3	1	1	2	0	7
Fruit	0	0	0	0	1	1
Starch	0	0	4	0	0	4
Fat	2 ½	2	0	2	3	9 ½

6 Meals Menu Plan

Macro	Meal 1	Meal 2	Meal 3	Meal 4	Meal 5	Meal 6	Total
Protein	4	3	4	4	6	3	24
Veggie	1	1	2	1	2	0	7
Fruit	0	0	0	0	0	1	1
Starch	0	4	0	0	0	0	4
Fat	2	0	1	1 ½	2	3	9 ½

Following are example menus for the weight loss formula covering resistance/weight training days for those in the 190 pound category. You may look at the Meal Chart to pick different foods that suit your taste buds.

Example Menus

Strenuous Days

190 lbs.

5 Meals Plan

Breakfast Omelette made with 1 whole Omega-3 egg, 5 egg whites, 4 slices low-sodium turkey bacon, 2 Tbs. sun-dried tomatoes, ½ cup chopped onions, ¾ cup sliced mushrooms & 1-½ oz. Feta cheese; green tea

Lunch: 6 oz. tuna mixed with 2 Tbs. EVOO mayo on top of a bed of Romaine, 1 cup sliced cucumbers & 1 cup sliced tomatoes

Post-Workout Snack: 1 sandwich made with gluten-free or Ezekiel bread (2 slices) with 4-½ oz. turkey slices topped with 1 large thick slice of onion & tomato & 2 large thick slices of green bell pepper

Dinner: 6-½ oz. grilled chicken breast cooked in 1 tsp. EVOO, 1-½ cups cooked kale with 1 tsp. butter & hot sauce

Bedtime Snack: 1-⅓ scoop low-carb chocolate protein powder mixed with ⅓ cup blueberries, 3 Tbs. almond slivers & enough pure almond milk to make pudding consistency

6 Meals Plan

Breakfast: 1-⅓ cup tofu cooked in 2 tsp. EVOO; 1 cup sliced cucumbers, ½ cup sliced tomatoes & ¼ cup sliced onions made into a salad with a little vinegar & Stevia ; 1 cup green tea

Post-Workout Snack: 3 oz. grilled chicken breast, 8 oz. sweet potato & ⅔ cup green beans

Lunch: 4 oz. grilled chicken breast, 1-⅓ cup green beans topped with 1 tsp. butter

Snack: 1 cup low-fat cottage cheese mixed with 6 cherry tomatoes & 1-½ Tbs. chia seeds

Dinner: 6 oz. lean roast beef, 1 cup cooked cabbage & 6 baby carrots topped with 2 tsp. butter

Bedtime Snack: 1 scoop low-carb protein powder mixed with 8 oz. pure almond milk; 5 large strawberries sliced and mixed with 3 Tbs. crumbled walnuts

Strenuous Days Blueprint

Protein: 25 blocks

Veggies: 7.5 blocks

Fruits: 1 block

Starches: 4

Fats: 10 blocks

STRENUOUS DAYS – 200 lbs.

The weight loss formula for resistance/weight training days includes healthy proteins, vegetables, fruits, and essential fats. We will also add starches as your body will need to replenish glycogen and recharge your metabolism. This blueprint should be used 1-2 times per week.

5 Meals Menu Plan

Macro	Meal 1	Meal 2	Meal 3	Meal 4	Meal 5	Total
Protein	5	4	5	7	4	25
Veggie	3	1 ½	1	2	0	7 ½
Fruit	0	0	0	0	1	1
Starch	0	0	4	0	0	4
Fat	3	2	0	2	3	10

6 Meals Menu Plan

Macro	Meal 1	Meal 2	Meal 3	Meal 4	Meal 5	Meal 6	Total
Protein	4	4	4	4	6	3	25
Veggie	1 ½	1	2	1	2	0	7 ½
Fruit	0	0	0	0	0	1	1
Starch	0	4	0	0	0	0	4
Fat	2	0	1	2	2	3	10

Following are example menus for the weight loss formula covering resistance/weight training days for those in the 200 pound category. You may look at the Meal Chart to pick different foods that suit your taste buds.

<u>**Example Menus**</u>

Strenuous Days

200 lbs.

5 Meals Plan

Breakfast Omelette made with 2 whole Omega-3 egg, 4 egg whites, 4 slices low-sodium turkey bacon, 2 Tbs. sun-dried tomatoes, ½ cup chopped onions & 1 oz. Feta cheese; green tea

Lunch: 6 oz. tuna mixed with 2 Tbs. EVOO mayo on top of a bed of Romaine, 1 cup sliced cucumbers, ¼ cup sliced onions & 1 cup sliced tomatoes

Post-Workout Snack: 1 sandwich made with gluten-free or Ezekiel bread (2 slices) with 5 oz. turkey slices topped with 1 large thick slice of onion & tomato & 2 large thick slices of green bell pepper

Dinner: 7 oz. grilled chicken breast cooked in 1 tsp. EVOO, 1-½ cups cooked kale with 1 tsp. butter & hot sauce

Bedtime Snack: 1-⅓ scoop low-carb chocolate protein powder mixed with ⅓ cup blueberries, 3 Tbs. almond slivers & enough pure almond milk to make pudding consistency

6 Meals Plan

Breakfast: 1-⅓ cup tofu cooked in 2 tsp. EVOO; 1 sliced cucumbers, 6 cherry tomatoes & ¼ cup sliced onions made into a salad with a little vinegar & Stevia ; 1 cup green tea

Post-Workout Snack: 4 oz. grilled chicken breast, 8 oz. sweet potato & ⅔ cup green beans

Lunch: 4 oz. grilled chicken breast, 1-⅓ cup green beans topped with 1 tsp. butter

Snack: 1 cup low-fat cottage cheese mixed with 6 cherry tomatoes & 2 Tbs. chia seeds

Dinner: 6 oz. lean roast beef, 1 cup cooked cabbage & 6 baby carrots topped with 2 tsp. butter

Bedtime Snack: 1 scoop low-carb protein powder mixed with 8 oz. pure almond milk; 5 large strawberries sliced and mixed with 3 Tbs. crumbled walnuts

Strenuous Days Blueprint

Protein: 26 blocks

Veggies: 8 blocks

Fruits: 1 block

Starches: 4.5 blocks

Fats: 10.5 blocks

STRENUOUS DAYS – 210 lbs.

The weight loss formula for resistance/weight training days includes healthy proteins, vegetables, fruits, and essential fats. We will also add starches as your body will need to replenish glycogen and recharge your metabolism. This blueprint should be used 1-2 times per week.

5 Meals Menu Plan

Macro	Meal 1	Meal 2	Meal 3	Meal 4	Meal 5	Total
Protein	5	4	5	7	5	26
Veggie	3	2	1	2	0	8
Fruit	0	0	0	0	1	1
Starch	0	0	4 ½	0	0	4 ½
Fat	3	2	0	2 ½	3	10 ½

6 Meals Menu Plan

Macro	Meal 1	Meal 2	Meal 3	Meal 4	Meal 5	Meal 6	Total
Protein	4	4	4	4	6	4	26
Veggie	2	1	2	1	2	0	8
Fruit	0	0	0	0	0	1	1
Starch	0	4 ½	0	0	0	0	4 ½
Fat	2	0	1 ½	2	2	3	10 ½

Following are example menus for the weight loss formula covering resistance/weight training days for those in the 210 pound category. You may look at the Meal Chart to pick different foods that suit your taste buds.

5 Meals Plan

Breakfast Omelette made with 2 whole Omega-3 egg, 4 egg whites, 4 slices low-sodium turkey bacon, 2 Tbs. sun-dried tomatoes, ½ cup chopped onions, ¾ cup sliced mushrooms & 1 oz. Feta cheese; green tea

Lunch: 6 oz. tuna mixed with 2 Tbs. EVOO mayo on top of a bed of Romaine, 1 cup sliced cucumbers, ½ cup sliced onions & 1 cup sliced tomatoes

Post-Workout Snack: 1 sandwich made with gluten-free or Ezekiel bread (2 slices) with 5 oz. turkey slices topped with 1 large thick slice of onion & tomato & 2 large thick slices of green bell pepper; ¼ cup oats on side

Dinner: 7 oz. grilled chicken breast cooked in 1 tsp. EVOO, 1-½ cups cooked kale with 1-½ tsp. butter & hot sauce

Bedtime Snack: 1-⅔ scoop low-carb chocolate protein powder mixed with ⅓ cup blueberries, 3 Tbs. almond slivers & enough pure almond milk to make pudding consistency

6 Meals Plan

Breakfast: 1-⅓ cup tofu cooked in 2 tsp. EVOO; 1 cup sliced cucumbers, 9 cherry tomatoes & ¼ cup sliced onions made into a salad with a little vinegar & Stevia ; 1 cup green tea

Post-Workout Snack: 4 oz. grilled chicken breast, 9 oz. sweet potato & ⅔ cup green beans

Lunch: 4 oz. grilled chicken breast, 1-⅓ cup green beans topped with 1-½ tsp. butter

Snack: 1 cup low-fat cottage cheese mixed with 6 cherry tomatoes & 2 Tbs. chia seeds

Dinner: 6 oz. lean roast beef, 1 cup cooked cabbage & 6 baby carrots topped with 2 tsp. butter

Bedtime Snack: 1-⅓ scoops low-carb protein powder mixed with 8 oz. pure almond milk; 5 large strawberries sliced and mixed with 3 Tbs. crumbled walnuts

Strenuous Days Blueprint

Protein: 27.5 blocks

Veggies: 8 blocks

Fruits: 1 block

Starches: 4.5

Fats: 11 blocks

STRENUOUS DAYS – 220 lbs.

The weight loss formula for resistance/weight training days includes healthy proteins, vegetables, fruits, and essential fats. We will also add starches as your body will need to replenish glycogen and recharge your metabolism. This blueprint should be used 1-2 times per week.

5 Meals Menu Plan

Macro	Meal 1	Meal 2	Meal 3	Meal 4	Meal 5	Total
Protein	5 ½	5	5	7	5	27 ½
Veggie	3	2	1	2	0	8
Fruit	0	0	0	0	1	1
Starch	0	0	4 ½	0	0	4 ½
Fat	3	2	0	3	3	11

6 Meals Menu Plan

Macro	Meal 1	Meal 2	Meal 3	Meal 4	Meal 5	Meal 6	Total
Protein	4	5	4 ½	4	6	4	27 ½
Veggie	2	1	2	1	2	0	8
Fruit	0	0	0	0	0	1	1
Starch	0	4 ½	0	0	0	0	4 ½
Fat	2	0	2	2	2	3	11

Following are example menus for the weight loss formula covering resistance/weight training days for those in the 220 pound category. You may look at the Meal Chart to pick different foods that suit your taste buds.

5 Meals Plan

Breakfast Omelette made with 2 whole Omega-3 egg, 4 egg whites, 5 slices low-sodium turkey bacon, 2 Tbs. sun-dried tomatoes, ½ cup chopped onions, ¾ cup sliced mushrooms & 1 oz. Feta cheese; green tea

Lunch: 7-½ oz. tuna mixed with 2 Tbs. EVOO mayo on top of a bed of Romaine, 1 cup sliced cucumbers, ½ cup sliced onions & 1 cup sliced tomatoes

Post-Workout Snack: 1 sandwich made with gluten-free or Ezekiel bread (2 slices) with 5 oz. turkey slices topped with 1 large thick slice of onion & tomato & 2 large thick slices of green bell pepper; ¼ cup oats on side

Dinner: 7 oz. grilled chicken breast cooked in 1 tsp. EVOO, 1-½ cups cooked kale with 2 tsp. butter & hot sauce

Bedtime Snack: 1-⅔ scoop low-carb chocolate protein powder mixed with ⅓ cup blueberries, 3 Tbs. almond slivers & enough pure almond milk to make pudding consistency

6 Meals Plan

Breakfast: 1-⅓ cup tofu cooked in 2 tsp. EVOO; 1 cup sliced cucumbers, 9 cherry tomatoes & ¼ cup sliced onions made into a salad with a little vinegar & Stevia ; 1 cup green tea

Post-Workout Snack: 5 oz. grilled chicken breast, 9 oz. sweet potato & ⅔ cup green beans

Lunch: 4-½ oz. grilled chicken breast, 1-⅓ cup green beans topped with 2 tsp. butter

Snack: 1 cup low-fat cottage cheese mixed with 6 cherry tomatoes & 2 Tbs. chia seeds

Dinner: 6 oz. lean roast beef, 1 cup cooked cabbage & 6 baby carrots topped with 2 tsp. butter

Bedtime Snack: 1-⅓ scoops low-carb protein powder mixed with 8 oz. pure almond milk; 5 large strawberries sliced and mixed with 3 Tbs. crumbled walnuts

Strenuous Days Blueprint

Protein: 29 blocks

Veggies: 8.5 blocks

Fruits: 1 block

Starches: 4.5 blocks

Fats: 11.5 blocks

STRENUOUS DAYS – 230 lbs.

The weight loss formula for resistance/weight training days includes healthy proteins, vegetables, fruits, and essential fats. We will also add starches as your body will need to replenish glycogen and recharge your metabolism. This blueprint should be used 1-2 times per week.

5 Meals Menu Plan						
Macro	Meal 1	Meal 2	Meal 3	Meal 4	Meal 5	Total
Protein	6	5	6	7	5	29
Veggie	3	2	1	2 ½	0	8 ½
Fruit	0	0	0	0	1	1
Starch	0	0	4 ½	0	0	4 ½
Fat	3	2 ½	0	3	3	11 ½

6 Meals Menu Plan							
Macro	Meal 1	Meal 2	Meal 3	Meal 4	Meal 5	Meal 6	Total
Protein	5	5	5	4	6	4	29
Veggie	2	1	2	1 ½	2	0	8 ½
Fruit	0	0	0	0	0	1	1
Starch	0	4 ½	0	0	0	0	4 ½
Fat	2	0	2	2	2	3 ½	11 ½

Following are example menus for the weight loss formula covering resistance/weight training days for those in the 230 pound category. You may look at the Meal Chart to pick different foods that suit your taste buds.

5 Meals Plan

Breakfast Omelette made with 2 whole Omega-3 egg, 6 egg whites, 4 slices low-sodium turkey bacon, 2 Tbs. sun-dried tomatoes, ½ cup chopped onions, ¾ cup sliced mushrooms & 1 oz. Feta cheese; green tea

Lunch: 7-½ oz. tuna mixed with 1-½ Tbs. EVOO mayo on top of a bed of Romaine, 1 cup sliced cucumbers, ½ cup sliced onions & 1 cup sliced tomatoes drizzled with 1 tsp. flaxseed oil

Post-Workout Snack: 1 sandwich made with gluten-free or Ezekiel bread (2 slices) with 6 oz. turkey slices topped with 1 large thick slice of onion & tomato & 2 large thick slices of green bell pepper; ¼ cup oats on side

Dinner: 7 oz. grilled chicken breast cooked in 1 tsp. EVOO, ¾ cup cooked kale w/1 tsp. butter & hot sauce; side salad w/ Romaine lettuce, 6 cherry tomatoes, 3 chopped baby carrots & ¼ cup sliced cucumbers w/1 tsp. EVOO

Bedtime Snack: 1-⅔ scoop low-carb chocolate protein powder mixed with ⅓ cup blueberries, 3 Tbs. almond slivers & enough pure almond milk to make pudding consistency

6 Meals Plan

Breakfast: 1 cup tofu & 3 oz. salmon cooked in 2 tsp. EVOO; 1 cup sliced cucumbers, 9 cherry tomatoes & ¼ cup sliced onions made into a salad with a little vinegar & Stevia ; 1 cup green tea

Post-Workout Snack: 5 oz. grilled chicken breast, 9 oz. sweet potato & ⅔ cup green beans

Lunch: 5 oz. grilled chicken breast, 1-⅓ cup green beans topped with 2 tsp. butter

Snack: 1 cup low-fat cottage cheese mixed with 9 cherry tomatoes & 2 Tbs. chia seeds

Dinner: 6 oz. lean roast beef, 1 cup cooked cabbage & 6 baby carrots topped with 2 tsp. butter

Bedtime Snack: 1-⅓ scoops low-carb protein powder mixed with 8 oz. pure almond milk; 5 large strawberries sliced and mixed with 3-½ Tbs. crumbled walnuts

Strenuous Days Blueprint
Protein: 30 blocks
Veggies: 9 blocks
Fruits: 1 block
Starches: 5 blocks
Fats: 12 blocks

STRENUOUS DAYS – 240 lbs.

The weight loss formula for resistance/weight training days includes healthy proteins, vegetables, fruits, and essential fats. We will also add starches as your body will need to replenish glycogen and recharge your metabolism. This blueprint should be used 1-2 times per week.

5 Meals Menu Plan

Macro	Meal 1	Meal 2	Meal 3	Meal 4	Meal 5	Total
Protein	6	5	6	8	5	30
Veggie	3	2	1	3	0	9
Fruit	0	0	0	0	1	1
Starch	0	0	5	0	0	5
Fat	3	3	0	3	3	12

6 Meals Menu Plan

Macro	Meal 1	Meal 2	Meal 3	Meal 4	Meal 5	Meal 6	Total
Protein	5	5	5	4	7	4	30
Veggie	2	1	2	2	2	0	9
Fruit	0	0	0	0	0	1	1
Starch	0	5	0	0	0	0	5
Fat	2	0	2	2	2	4	12

Following are example menus for the weight loss formula covering resistance/weight training days for those in the 240 pound category. You may look at the Meal Chart to pick different foods that suit your taste buds.

Example Menus

Strenuous Days

240 lbs.

5 Meals Plan

Breakfast Omelette made with 2 whole Omega-3 egg, 6 egg whites, 4 slices low-sodium turkey bacon, 2 Tbs. sun-dried tomatoes, ½ cup chopped onions, ¾ cup sliced mushrooms & 1 oz. Feta cheese; green tea

Lunch: 7-½ oz. tuna mixed with 2 Tbs. EVOO mayo on top of a bed of Romaine, 1 cup sliced cucumbers, ½ cup sliced onions & 1 cup sliced tomatoes drizzled with 1 tsp. flaxseed oil

Post-Workout Snack: 1 sandwich made with gluten-free or Ezekiel bread (2 slices) with 6 oz. turkey slices topped with 1 large thick slice of onion & tomato & 2 large thick slices of green bell pepper; ½ cup oats on side

Dinner: 8 oz. grilled chicken breast cooked in 1 tsp. EVOO, ¾ cup cooked kale w/1 tsp. butter & hot sauce; side salad w/ Romaine lettuce, 6 cherry tomatoes, 6 chopped baby carrots & ½ cup sliced cucumbers w/1 tsp. EVOO

Bedtime Snack: 1-⅔ scoop low-carb chocolate protein powder mixed with ⅓ cup blueberries, 3 Tbs. almond slivers & enough pure almond milk to make pudding consistency

6 Meals Plan

Breakfast: 1 cup tofu & 3 oz. salmon cooked in 2 tsp. EVOO; 1 cup sliced cucumbers, 9 cherry tomatoes & ¼ cup sliced onions made into a salad with a little vinegar & Stevia ; 1 cup green tea

Post-Workout Snack: 5 oz. grilled chicken breast, 10 oz. sweet potato & ⅔ cup green beans

Lunch: 5 oz. grilled chicken breast, 1-⅓ cup green beans topped with 2 tsp. butter

Snack: 1 cup low-fat cottage cheese mixed with 9 cherry tomatoes, ½ cup chopped red bell pepper & 2 Tbs. chia seeds

Dinner: 7 oz. lean roast beef, 1 cup cooked cabbage & 6 baby carrots topped with 2 tsp. butter

Bedtime Snack: 1-⅓ scoops low-carb protein powder mixed with 8 oz. pure almond milk; 5 large strawberries sliced and mixed with 4 Tbs. crumbled walnuts

Strenuous Days Blueprint

Protein: 31 blocks

Veggies: 9.5 blocks

Fruits: 1 block

Starches: 5 blocks

Fats: 12.5 blocks

STRENUOUS DAYS – 250 lbs.

The weight loss formula for resistance/weight training days includes healthy proteins, vegetables, fruits, and essential fats. We will also add starches as your body will need to replenish glycogen and recharge your metabolism. This blueprint should be used 1-2 times per week.

5 Meals Menu Plan

Macro	Meal 1	Meal 2	Meal 3	Meal 4	Meal 5	Total
Protein	6	5	6	8	6	31
Veggie	3	2 ½	1	3	0	9 ½
Fruit	0	0	0	0	1	1
Starch	0	0	5	0	0	5
Fat	3	3	0	3	3 ½	12 ½

6 Meals Menu Plan

Macro	Meal 1	Meal 2	Meal 3	Meal 4	Meal 5	Meal 6	Total
Protein	5	5	5	4	7	5	31
Veggie	2	1	2	2	2 ½	0	9 ½
Fruit	0	0	0	0	0	1	1
Starch	0	5	0	0	0	0	5
Fat	2	0	2	2	2 ½	4	12 ½

Following are example menus for the weight loss formula covering resistance/weight training days for those in the 250 pound category. You may look at the Meal Chart to pick different foods that suit your taste buds.

5 Meals Plan

Breakfast Omelette made with 2 whole Omega-3 egg, 6 egg whites, 4 slices low-sodium turkey bacon, 2 Tbs. sun-dried tomatoes, ½ cup chopped onions, ¾ cup sliced mushrooms & 1 oz. Feta cheese; green tea

Lunch: 7-½ oz. tuna mixed with 2 Tbs. EVOO mayo on top of a bed of Romaine, ½ cup sliced onions, ½ cup sliced bell peppers & 1 cup sliced tomatoes drizzled with 1 tsp. flaxseed oil

Post-Workout Snack: 1 sandwich made with gluten-free or Ezekiel bread (2 slices) with 6 oz. turkey slices topped with 1 large thick slice of onion & tomato & 2 large thick slices of green bell pepper; ½ cup oats on side

Dinner: 8 oz. grilled chicken breast cooked in 1 tsp. EVOO, ¾ cup cooked kale w/1 tsp. butter & hot sauce; side salad w/ Romaine lettuce, 6 cherry tomatoes, 6 chopped baby carrots & ½ cup sliced cucumbers w/1 tsp. EVOO

Bedtime Snack: 2 scoops low-carb chocolate protein powder mixed with ⅓ cup blueberries, 3-½ Tbs. almond slivers & enough pure almond milk to make pudding consistency

6 Meals Plan

Breakfast: 1 cup tofu & 3 oz. salmon cooked in 2 tsp. EVOO; 1 cup sliced cucumbers, 9 cherry tomatoes & ¼ cup sliced onions made into a salad with a little vinegar & Stevia ; 1 cup green tea

Post-Workout Snack: 5 oz. grilled chicken breast, 10 oz. sweet potato & ⅔ cup green beans

Lunch: 5 oz. grilled chicken breast, 1-⅓ cup green beans topped with 2 tsp. butter

Snack: 1 cup low-fat cottage cheese mixed with 9 cherry tomatoes, ½ cup chopped red bell pepper & 2 Tbs. chia seeds

Dinner: 7 oz. lean roast beef, 1 cup cooked cabbage & 9 baby carrots topped with 2-½ tsp. butter

Bedtime Snack: 1-⅔ scoops low-carb protein powder mixed with 8 oz. pure almond milk; 5 large strawberries sliced and mixed with 4 Tbs. crumbled walnuts

Strenuous Days Blueprint
Protein: 32.5 blocks
Veggies: 10 blocks
Fruits: 1 block
Starches: 5.5 blocks
Fats: 13 blocks

STRENUOUS DAYS – 260 lbs.

The weight loss formula for resistance/weight training days includes healthy proteins, vegetables, fruits, and essential fats. We will also add starches as your body will need to replenish glycogen and recharge your metabolism. This blueprint should be used 1-2 times per week.

5 Meals Menu Plan

Macro	Meal 1	Meal 2	Meal 3	Meal 4	Meal 5	Total
Protein	6	6	6	8 ½	6	32 ½
Veggie	3	3	1	3	0	10
Fruit	0	0	0	0	1	1
Starch	0	0	5 ½	0	0	5 ½
Fat	3	3	0	3	4	13

6 Meals Menu Plan

Macro	Meal 1	Meal 2	Meal 3	Meal 4	Meal 5	Meal 6	Total
Protein	5	5	5	4	8 ½	5	32 ½
Veggie	2	1	2	2	3	0	10
Fruit	0	0	0	0	0	1	1
Starch	0	5 ½	0	0	0	0	5 ½
Fat	2	0	2	2 ½	2 ½	4	13

Following are example menus for the weight loss formula covering resistance/weight training days for those in the 260 pound category. You may look at the Meal Chart to pick different foods that suit your taste buds.

5 Meals Plan

Breakfast Omelette made with 2 whole Omega-3 egg, 6 egg whites, 4 slices low-sodium turkey bacon, 2 Tbs. sun-dried tomatoes, ½ cup chopped onions, ¾ cup sliced mushrooms & 1 oz. Feta cheese; green tea

Lunch: 9 oz. tuna mixed with 1-½ Tbs. EVOO mayo on top of a bed of Romaine, ½ cup sliced onions, 1 cup sliced bell peppers & 1 cup sliced tomatoes drizzled with 1-½ tsp. flaxseed oil

Post-Workout Snack: 1 sandwich made with gluten-free or Ezekiel bread (2 slices) with 6 oz. turkey slices topped with 1 large thick slice of onion & tomato & 2 large thick slices of green bell pepper; ¾ cup oats on side

Dinner: 8-½ oz. grilled chicken breast cooked in 1 tsp. EVOO, ¾ cup cooked kale w/1 tsp. butter & hot sauce; side salad w/ Romaine lettuce, 6 cherry tomatoes, 6 chopped baby carrots & ½ cup sliced cucumbers w/1 tsp. EVOO

Bedtime Snack: 2 scoops low-carb chocolate protein powder mixed with ⅓ cup blueberries, 4 Tbs. almond slivers & enough pure almond milk to make pudding consistency

6 Meals Plan

Breakfast: 1 cup tofu & 3 oz. salmon cooked in 2 tsp. EVOO; 1 cup sliced cucumbers, 9 cherry tomatoes & ¼ cup sliced onions made into a salad with a little vinegar & Stevia ; 1 cup green tea

Post-Workout Snack: 5 oz. grilled chicken breast, 11 oz. sweet potato & ⅔ cup green beans

Lunch: 5 oz. grilled chicken breast, 1-⅓ cup green beans topped with 2 tsp. butter

Snack: 1 cup low-fat cottage cheese mixed with 9 cherry tomatoes, ½ cup chopped red bell pepper & 2-½ Tbs. chia seeds

Dinner: 8-½ oz. lean roast beef, 1 cup cooked cabbage & 12 baby carrots topped with 2-½ tsp. butter

Bedtime Snack: 1-⅔ scoops low-carb protein powder mixed with 8 oz. pure almond milk; 5 large strawberries sliced and mixed with 4 Tbs. crumbled walnuts

Strenuous Days Blueprint

Protein: 34 blocks

Veggies: 10 blocks

Fruits: 1.5 blocks

Starches: 5.5 blocks

Fats: 13.5 blocks

STRENUOUS DAYS – 270 lbs.

The weight loss formula for resistance/weight training days includes healthy proteins, vegetables, fruits, and essential fats. We will also add starches as your body will need to replenish glycogen and recharge your metabolism. This blueprint should be used 1-2 times per week.

5 Meals Menu Plan

Macro	Meal 1	Meal 2	Meal 3	Meal 4	Meal 5	Total
Protein	6	6	6	8 ½	7 ½	34
Veggie	3	3	1	3	0	10
Fruit	0	0	0	0	1 ½	1 ½
Starch	0	0	5 ½	0	0	5 ½
Fat	3	3	0	3 ½	4	13 ½

6 Meals Menu Plan

Macro	Meal 1	Meal 2	Meal 3	Meal 4	Meal 5	Meal 6	Total
Protein	5	6 ½	5	4	8 ½	5	34
Veggie	2	1	2	2	3	0	10
Fruit	0	0	0	0	0	1 ½	1 ½
Starch	0	5 ½	0	0	0	0	5 ½
Fat	2	0	2	3	2 ½	4	13 ½

Following are example menus for the weight loss formula covering resistance/weight training days for those in the 270 pound category. You may look at the Meal Chart to pick different foods that suit your taste buds.

5 Meals Plan

Breakfast Omelette made with 2 whole Omega-3 egg, 6 egg whites, 4 slices low-sodium turkey bacon, 2 Tbs. sun-dried tomatoes, ½ cup chopped onions, ¾ cup sliced mushrooms & 1 oz. Feta cheese; green tea

Lunch: 9 oz. tuna mixed with 1-½ Tbs. EVOO mayo on top of a bed of Romaine, ½ cup sliced onions, 1 cup sliced bell peppers & 1 cup sliced tomatoes drizzled with 1-½ tsp. flaxseed oil

Post-Workout Snack: 1 sandwich made with gluten-free or Ezekiel bread (2 slices) with 6 oz. turkey slices topped with 1 large thick slice of onion & tomato & 2 large thick slices of green bell pepper; ¾ cup oats on side

Dinner: 8-½ oz. grilled chicken breast cooked in 1 tsp. EVOO, ¾ cup cooked kale w/1 tsp. butter & hot sauce; side salad w/ Romaine lettuce, 6 cherry tomatoes, 6 chopped baby carrots & 1 cup sliced bell peppers with 1-½ tsp. EVOO

Bedtime Snack: 2 scoops low-carb chocolate protein powder mixed with water; ⅓ cup low-fat cottage cheese mixed with ⅓ cup blueberries & 4 Tbs. almond slivers

6 Meals Plan

Breakfast: 1 cup tofu & 3 oz. salmon cooked in 2 tsp. EVOO; 1 cup sliced cucumbers, 9 cherry tomatoes & ¼ cup sliced onions made into a salad with a little vinegar & Stevia ; 1 cup green tea

Post-Workout Snack: 6-½ oz. grilled chicken breast, 11 oz. sweet potato, ⅔ cup green beans

Lunch: 5 oz. grilled chicken breast, 1-⅓ cup green beans topped with 2 tsp. butter

Snack: 1 cup low-fat cottage cheese mixed with 9 cherry tomatoes, ½ cup chopped red bell pepper & 3 Tbs. chia seeds

Dinner: 8-½ oz. lean roast beef, 1 cup cooked cabbage & 12 baby carrots topped with 2-½ tsp. butter

Bedtime Snack: 1-⅔ scoops low-carb protein powder mixed with 8 oz. pure almond milk; 7-8 large strawberries sliced and mixed with 4 Tbs. crumbled walnuts

Strenuous Days Blueprint

Protein: 35 blocks

Veggies: 10 blocks

Fruits: 1.5 blocks

Starches: 6 blocks

Fats: 14 blocks

STRENUOUS DAYS – 280 lbs.

The weight loss formula for resistance/weight training days includes healthy proteins, vegetables, fruits, and essential fats. We will also add starches as your body will need to replenish glycogen and recharge your metabolism. This blueprint should be used 1-2 times per week.

5 Meals Menu Plan

Macro	Meal 1	Meal 2	Meal 3	Meal 4	Meal 5	Total
Protein	6	6	7	8 ½	7 ½	35
Veggie	3	3	1	3	0	10
Fruit	0	0	0	0	1 ½	1 ½
Starch	0	0	6	0	0	6
Fat	3	3	0	3 ½	4 ½	14

6 Meals Menu Plan

Macro	Meal 1	Meal 2	Meal 3	Meal 4	Meal 5	Meal 6	Total
Protein	5	6 ½	6	4	8 ½	5	35
Veggie	2	1	2	2	3	0	10
Fruit	0	0	0	0	0	1 ½	1 ½
Starch	0	6	0	0	0	0	6
Fat	2	0	2	3	2 ½	4 ½	14

Following are example menus for the weight loss formula covering resistance/weight training days for those in the 280 pound category. You may look at the Meal Chart to pick different foods that suit your taste buds.

Example Menus

Strenuous Days

280 lbs.

5 Meals Plan

Breakfast Omelette made with 2 whole Omega-3 egg, 6 egg whites, 4 slices low-sodium turkey bacon, 2 Tbs. sun-dried tomatoes, ½ cup chopped onions, ¾ cup sliced mushrooms & 1 oz. Feta cheese; green tea

Lunch: 9 oz. tuna mixed with 1-½ Tbs. EVOO mayo on top of a bed of Romaine, ½ cup sliced onions, 1 cup sliced bell peppers & 1 cup sliced tomatoes drizzled with 1-½ tsp. flaxseed oil

Post-Workout Snack: 1-½ sandwiches made with gluten-free or Ezekiel bread (3 slices) with 7 oz. turkey slices topped with 1 large thick slice of onion & tomato & 2 large thick slices of green bell pepper

Dinner: 8-½ oz. grilled chicken breast cooked in 1 tsp. EVOO, ¾ cup cooked kale w/1 tsp. butter & hot sauce; side salad w/ Romaine lettuce, 6 cherry tomatoes, 6 chopped baby carrots & 1 cup sliced bell peppers with 1-½ tsp. EVOO

Bedtime Snack: 2 scoops low-carb chocolate protein powder mixed with water; ⅓ cup low-fat cottage cheese mixed with ⅓ cup blueberries & 4-½ Tbs. almond slivers

6 Meals Plan

Breakfast: 1 cup tofu & 3 oz. salmon cooked in 2 tsp. EVOO; 1 cup sliced cucumbers, 9 cherry tomatoes & ¼ cup sliced onions made into a salad with a little vinegar & Stevia ; 1 cup green tea

Post-Workout Snack: 6-½ oz. grilled chicken breast, 12 oz. sweet potato, ⅔ cup green beans

Lunch: 6 oz. grilled chicken breast, 1-⅓ cup green beans topped with 2 tsp. butter

Snack: 1 cup low-fat cottage cheese mixed with 9 cherry tomatoes, ½ cup chopped red bell pepper & 3 Tbs. chia seeds

Dinner: 8-½ oz. lean roast beef, 1 cup cooked cabbage & 12 baby carrots topped with 2-½ tsp. butter

Bedtime Snack: 1-⅔ scoops low-carb protein powder mixed with 8 oz. pure almond milk; 7-8 large strawberries sliced and mixed with 4-½ Tbs. crumbled walnuts

11 – Transition & Manage Your Goals

What you will learn in this section:
- ✓ How to transition after goals are reached.
- ✓ How to plan meals after transitioning.

Transition Nutrition

Now that you have reached your goals, you will need to transition so that you can maintain your body weight. Over the past several weeks, months, or years, you have allowed your body to become accustomed to running on an energy deficit. Failing to transition effectively can cause many issues from digestive problems to regaining body weight. This is something you don't want, so you will need to allow your body to shift from the extreme fat loss process to the maintenance process.

You will continue to cycle calories and carbohydrates depending on your day's activity. For instance, you will still eat less calories and carbohydrates on rest days. You'll also increase calories and carbohydrates on more active days. That part of the plan has not changed as you still want to continue feeding your body as is necessary. To transition, you will increase both calories and carbohydrates for 14 to 28 days before leveling out for your maintenance weight.

The change process is actually quite simple:

➢ Rest & Active Recovery Days → become Normal Workout Days
➢ Normal Workout Days → become Strenuous Workout Days
➢ Strenuous Workout Days → add 50 percent more carbohydrates (i.e., vegetables, fruits, and starches)

You are going to completely throw out your menu plans for rest and activity recovery days. Your transition menu plan for these days will now include your normal workout day menu plan. Your previous normal workout menu plan will also be replaced by your previous menu plans for strenuous workout days. Fine tuning will come into play with the new strenuous workout days where you will add 50 percent more vegetable, fruit, and starchy carbohydrates. As you will see below, the total carbohydrate counts for the 160 pound menu plan is 5.5 veggies, 1 fruit, and 3.5 starches. To increase these counts by 50 percent, you just add "half" of each amount to the current totals. Your new totals will include 8.25 veggies, 1.5 fruit, and 5.25 starches. Don't worry so much about the technicalities of the fractions. You may round down to 8 veggie blocks and 5 starch blocks.

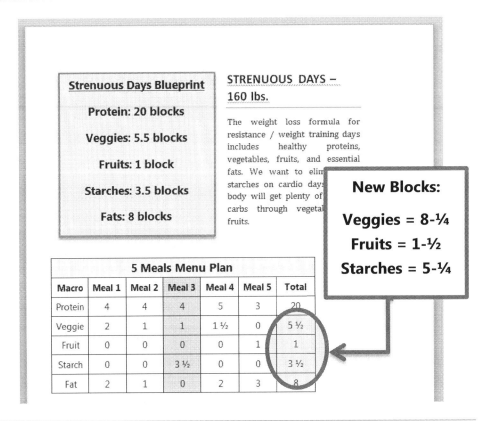

You will be adding approximately 175 calories for this 160 pound menu plan on the new strenuous workout days. If you think this is too much of an immediate increase, add half for the first few days or week. Then increase a bit more until you've reached the transition menu numbers and continue for 14 to 28 days.

Maintenance Nutrition

Maintenance nutrition is a bit tricky, and you will have to adjust little by little until you find your body's comfort zone. There are no two people alike. Everybody has a different composition, has different metabolic rates, and use different energy levels depending on activity. You may increase carbohydrates by one block at a time for one to two weeks and see how your body is adjusting. If you find that you are continually losing weight, then you know you have room to increase further. When you find that you are gaining, you will know you need to cut back. Pay close attention to your scale weight and girth measurements during this time to keep you on track.

12 – Meal Charts

What you will learn in this section:

✓ What foods belong to each food group: protein, carbohydrate, and fat.

✓ What carbohydrate foods belong to each carbohydrate group: vegetable, fruit, and starch.

✓ What a block size is for each food using the formulas given in the phases given (Phase 3 and the transition phase).

Categories of Meal Charts Included

➢ Protein
➢ Vegetables
➢ Fruits
➢ Starches
➢ Fat
➢ FREE Foods

Phase 1 and 2 Meal Planners

For phase 1 and 2, you may use the meal charts to help you determine what foods are healthy. Do not worry so much about the block sizes. Just work on getting into the groove of eating healthy foods.

Phase 3 Meal Planners

For Phase 3 dieters – use the meal charts to personalize your own meal plans with these nutritional food items. Each food block item listed within each chart is equivalent to all other food block items. For instance, a protein choice of one ounce of lean beef is equivalent to one ounce of chicken or pork. It is also equivalent to two ounces of shrimp or 1.5 ounces of fish. For the fruit food blocks, seven cherries is equivalent to five large strawberries or one-third cup of blueberries. For equivalency, make sure you are exchanging the same food choices – protein for protein, fruit for fruit, etc.

A Note on Inflammatory Foods

The charts are extensive and cover most natural foods that you may want to include in your meals. Any foods that have more than a minor effect of inflammation on the body is not included as inflammation damages the body with disease and even makes you hold onto body fat, something you do not want. There are a few fruit items (i.e., dried cranberries, dates, and raisins) that are slightly inflammatory. They are starred on the chart. Because you will be eating a good amount of vegetables, you will be offsetting any effects these fruits may have. However, try to limit your intake of these particular fruits to one block per day. If for example you have two fruit blocks on your daily menu, you may choose one of the three starred fruit items for one of those blocks such as raisins. For the second block, have a non-starred fruit item such as an apple or grapefruit.

If there is a food that you really enjoy but is not on the list, you may email abby@911BodyResQ.com or https://www.facebook.com/Abby.911BodyResQ to ask whether it is a healthy food item and what the serving size is for it. If it's not considered healthy or natural, it will be considered one of your "treats."

Organic and Non-GMO Foods

Some foods such as soy, whole grains, and other produce have been genetically modified. As discussed in Chapter 5, genetically modified organisms (GMOs) are hazardous to health. Therefore, you want to opt for organic certified foods as they are not allowed to be genetically modified. Foods you may want to especially be careful with are whole grains such as barley, wheat, and rye. Also, be careful with dairy, potatoes, beets, squash, and papaya.

Protein Choices

Beef (lean) - 1 oz.
- Examples: flank steak, ground (95%), round steaks & tips, sirloin, roast

Bison - 1 oz.
- Examples: rib eye, round, roast, sirloin

Chicken - 1 oz.
- Examples: canned (no broth, low-sodium), breast, gizzards, liver

Deer (Venison) - 1 oz.
- Examples: ground, round, roast, tenderloin

Elk - 1 oz.
- Examples: roast, round, tenderloin

Pork - 1 oz.
- Examples: tenderloin

Seafood
- crab (Alaska or blue) - 2 oz.
- crab (dungeness or queen) - 1.5 oz.
- fish (i.e., salmon, mackerel, herring, tuna, sardines, etc.) - 1.5 oz.
- shrimp - 2 oz.
- NO artificial seafood

Turkey
- turkey bacon (low-sodium) - 2 slices
- turkey meat - 1 oz.

Veal - 1 oz.
- Examples: ground, sirloin

Other
- cottage cheese (low-fat 1-2%) - ¼ cup
- egg white - 2 large or 6 TBS.
- Greek yogurt - ⅓ cup
- natural deli meats (low sodium); NO packaged lunch meats
- protein powder or shake (low-carb) - ⅓ scoop of 20-25 gram scoop
- tempeh - 1.5 oz.
- tofu (firm) - ⅓ cup

Vegetable Choices

Vegetable	Qty
Artichokes, cooked	1
Asparagus, cooked	8 spears
Asparagus, raw	5 spears
Beets, cooked	½ cup
Broccoli, cooked	½ cup
Broccoli flowerets, raw	1-½ cups
Brussels Sprouts, cooked	½ cup
Cabbage, cooked	1 cup
Cabbage, raw	1-½ cups
Carrots, cooked	½ cup
Carrots (baby), raw	6 large
Cauliflower, cooked	1 cup
Cauliflower, raw	1 cup
Collards, cooked	½ cup
Eggplant, cooked	¾ cup
Green beans	¾ cup
Kale, cooked	¾ cup
Leeks, cooked/chopped	1 cup
Mushrooms, cooked	¾ cup
Mushrooms, raw	1-½ cups
Mustard Greens, cooked	1-½ cups
Okra, cooked	¾ cup
Onions, cooked	¼ cup

Vegetable	Qty
Onion, raw	½ cup
Pumpkin, cooked	⅔ cup
Radishes, sliced	1-½ cups
Salsa (low-sodium)	½ cup
Scallions	4 large
Sweet Peppers, cooked	½ cup
Sweet Peppers, raw	1 cup
Spinach, cooked	¾ cup
Squash-Butternut, cooked	⅓ cup
Squash-Spaghetti, cooked	⅔ cup
Sugar Snap Peas	2 oz.
Tomato, cooked	⅔ cup
Tomato, raw	1 cup
Tomato-Cherry/Grape	6
Tomato (crushed)	3.5 oz.
Tomato (sauce)	⅓ cup
Tomato (stewed)	½ cup
Tomato (sun-dried)	2 Tbs.
Tomato Juice (low sodium)	½ cup
Tomato Paste	2 Tbs.
Turnip Greens, cooked	1 cup
V8 Juice (low sodium)	½ cup
Zucchini, cooked	1 cup

Fruit Choices

Fruit	Qty	Fruit	Qty
Apple w/skin (2-½")	½	Mandarin Orange (2-¾")	½
Applesauce, unsweetened	⅓ cup	Mango, sliced	¼ cup
Apricots	2	Nectarine (2-⅓")	½
Banana (6")	½	Orange (2-5/8")	½
Blackberries	½ cup	Papaya, cubed	½ cup
Blueberries	⅓ cup	Peach (2-⅔")	½
Cantaloupe, cubed	½ cup	Pear, Asian (2-½")	½
Cherries, sweet	7	Pear, sliced	⅓ cup
*Cranberries, dried/sweet	1 Tbs.	Pineapple, diced	½ cup
Cranberries	⅔ cup	Plum (2-1/8")	1
*Date, deglet noor	1	Prune, unsweetened	1
Fig, raw	1	*Raisins, seedless/unpacked	1 Tbs.
Grapefruit (3-¾")	½	Raspberries	½ cup
Grapes, red or green	10	Strawberries, sliced	¾ cup
Honeydew	½ cup	Strawberries, large	5
Kiwi (3.2 oz.)	½	Tangerine (2-¾")	½
Lemon (2-3/8")	1	Watermelon, diced	¾ cup
Lime (2")	½		

Did you know?

Berries have been proven to reduce risk for everything from heart disease to memory loss and cancer? Fresh berries of all kinds are high in vitamin C, fiber, folic acid, and powerful phytonutrients. They are also delicious as they are nutritious!

Starch Choices

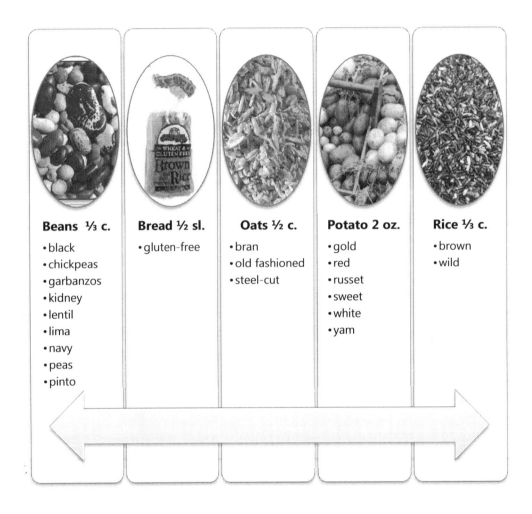

Beans ⅓ c.
- black
- chickpeas
- garbanzos
- kidney
- lentil
- lima
- navy
- peas
- pinto

Bread ½ sl.
- gluten-free

Oats ½ c.
- bran
- old fashioned
- steel-cut

Potato 2 oz.
- gold
- red
- russet
- sweet
- white
- yam

Rice ⅓ c.
- brown
- wild

Remember to get your starchy carbs in after a strenuous resistance or weight training workout! Your muscles will love you for it!

NOTE #1: Gluten-free bread can be purchased at natural food stores or at http://www.FoodForLife.com.

NOTE #2: Homemade or low-sodium commercially prepared hummus is also a starch you may opt for. One Tbs. is one serving.

Essential Fat Choices

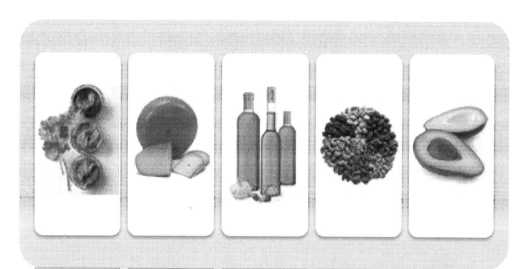

Butters (1 tsp.)	Cheese (1 oz. or ½ slice)	Oils (1 tsp.)	Nuts (1 TBS.)	Other
• almond	• blue	• avocado	• almonds	• avocado (¼ c.)
• butter	• cheddar	• coconut	• brazil	• chia seeds (1 TBS.)
• cashew	• colby jack	• extra virgin olive	• cashews	• coconut - shredded & unsweet (¼ c.)
• peanut	• feta	• fish	• flax seeds	• egg yolk (1)
• sesame	• gonda	• flaxseed	• hazelnuts	• EVOO mayo (1 TBS.)
• tahini	• monterey		• macadamia	• olives (1 oz.)
	• mozzarella		• pecans	
	• muenster		• pine nuts	
	• parmesan		• pistachios	
	• pepper jack		• pumpkin	
	• provolone		• sesame seeds	
	• string (½)		• sunflower seeds	
	• swiss		• walnuts	

Healthy Tip

Be sure to include plenty of essential fats in your menu. Those with Omega-3 fatty acids (i.e., flax seed, flaxseed oil, fish oil, chia seeds, and walnuts) are the most beneficial to your health and fat loss.

FREE Food Choices

The following list contains FREE foods. You may incorporate them into your menus with whatever quantity you prefer:

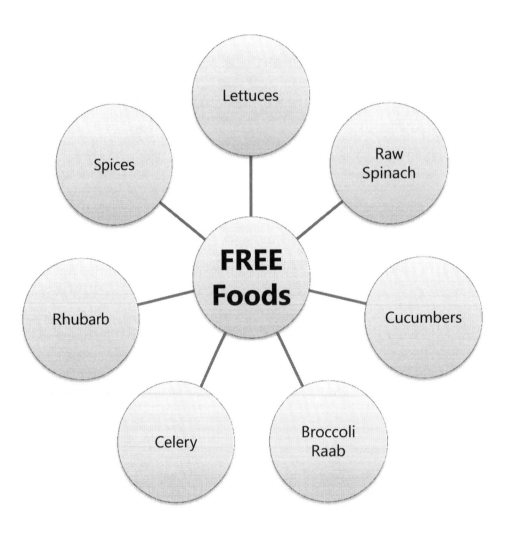

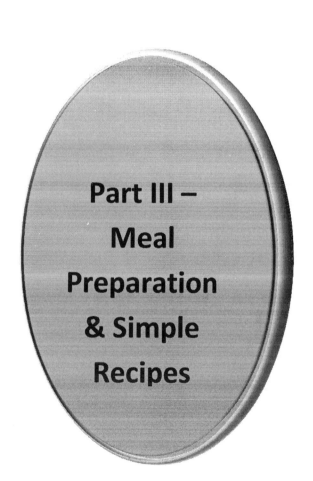

Part III –
Meal
Preparation
& Simple
Recipes

13 – Preparation is the Key to Success

What you will learn in this section:

✓ Planning your menu, grocery shopping, and meal preparation.
✓ Planning and preparation is the key to eating successfully.
✓ Investing in only useful kitchen utensils.

Let's face it! We live busy lives, and days of long preparing gourmet meals are over. Most people just don't have the time for it. Everyone wants quick and easy. Planning your meals is the key to staying on track. You need tasty and easy meals with variety that you can make day in and day out. Just make sure you are sticking to the 9 principles of healthy eating on a consistent basis.

To help you stick to the 9 principles of healthy eating, you will need to prepare your kitchen according to your plan. If the foods are not available, you will not succeed even if you do know what to eat. Stock your kitchen with healthy foods. Toss out the junk so that you will not be tempted by those empty calorie foods. After all, you may not notice that your unconscious pattern of behavior has made you guilty until after the fact. You can eliminate the feeling by staying on guard with planning and preparation.

Meal Planning for Phase 1 Users

Your first step is to clean out your kitchen! You will go through your refrigerator and pantry and get rid of all foods that are pre-packaged, processed, and refined. This will give you a clean slate with no temptations. For some of you, this will be difficult and you may need to work on only one or two habits at a time. Following are some helpful hints of what you could do when working on each habit:

> **Principle #3 – Melt Body Fat Like Crazy with Protein.** Rid all "meat-like" foods in your kitchen such as canned spam, Vienna sausages, hot dogs, Steak-ums, and other frozen processed meats. Also, throw away any flavored yogurts as most yogurts are full of additives like sugar, aspartame, and food coloring. Replace these items with fresh lean beef, skinless chicken or turkey breast, pork tenderloin, fish, and seafood. You may even include eggs, low-fat cottage cheese, and Greek yogurt. You'll find that mixing your cottage cheese and Greek yogurt with fresh fruit and nuts is much tastier, and it's much healthier as well. Greek yogurt also has a ton more protein than regular yogurt.

> **Principle #4 – Love Your Vegetables and Fruits.** Get rid of anything that resembles fruit such as canned vegetables and fruit, fruit cups, dried fruit, jams, and jellies as these are processed foods that cause inflammation. Replace these items with whole vegetables and fruits. Frozen vegetables are also fine as long as they aren't mixed with sauce and processed cheese.

> **Principle #5 – Meet Starchy Foods After the Gym Only.** This is probably the most difficult habit to build because many cultures have become accustomed to pre-packaged goods like bread, pasta, crackers, granola bars, rice cakes, etc. Note that these are the foods that have gotten two-thirds of Americans in trouble with their weight and health. Throw them out and replace them with whole foods such as old fashioned oatmeal, steel-cut oats, oat bran, brown rice, wild rice, potatoes, sweet potatoes, and quinoa. If you absolutely don't want to give up bread, then try Ezekiel bread or natural bread without gluten. You may check out Food for Life (http://www.FoodForLife.com/) to see where you can find this bread in your local area. Ezekiel bread contains no preservatives and only whole foods.

> **Principle #6 – Don't Allow Fat to be Your Enemy.** One of the worst foods you can put in your body is margarine because of the way it is

processed. Rodents won't even touch it because of the rancidity process it goes through prior to being marketed. Also, do away with unhealthy oils such as vegetable oil, canola oil, corn oil, safflower oil, soybean oil, and sunflower oil.[125] Replace these hydrogenated fats and oils with healthy fats like unsalted butter, coconut oil, extra virgin olive oil, flaxseed oil, flax seeds, chia seeds, walnuts, and avocados.

> **Principle #7 – Get Drunk with Water & Teas.** Gather and toss all the sugary and artificial drinks in your refrigerator such as juices, fruit punches, and sodas. Replace with pitchers of water and a variety of tea bags (i.e., black tea, green tea, white tea, and other herbal teas). Herbal tea bags come in many different types and flavors, and you can read their descriptions on their package to find out what each one is specifically used for. Some examples include: dandelion tea as a great diuretic, red clover tea for balancing women's hormones, and chamomile tea for calmness. Black, green, and white teas can be made by the pitcher as *iced tea* and sweetened with a natural herb called Stevia. Splenda is also okay. Other herbal teas can be made by individual cups.

> **Principle #8 – Have a Treat: Stick to the 90/10 Rule.** It may be difficult to stick to this principle if you have treats lying around the kitchen. Instead you may want to go out for your treats or stick a note on the treat with a date of when you can have it. The best way to stick to the 90/10 rule is by figuring how many meals and snacks you eat per week. Then figure what 10 percent of the total is. If you have five meals per day, that's 35 meals per week. Ten percent of 35 equates to 3.5 meals that you can treat yourself with. Mark your calendar with the date and meal that you will treat yourself. Just don't overdo your portions. Be sensible!

> **Principle #9 – Gain a New Favorite Hobby in Cooking.** Look at your calendar and set aside a certain amount of time per day or week, whether it is 30 minutes each day or 2.5 hours on Sundays. Look at simple cookbooks or magazines and get ideas of what you would enjoy eating. Then figure on a simple way of making those dishes. You will also find some basic foods in the next chapter that are easy to cook.

It's time to go shopping! Get familiar with where the healthiest food items are. Before you know it, you'll be navigating the grocery store like a pro! Shop as efficiently as possible, and reduce temptations and distractions so that you'll be sure to stock up on only healthy foods. Most grocery stores are laid out the same way with all the healthy, natural foods on the outside perimeter: produce (vegetables and fruit), proteins (beef, chicken, turkey, pork tenderloin, fish, and other seafood), and eggs and dairy (cottage cheese and Greek yogurt). Following is a basic list of foods that you can start with. Please be sure to check the meal charts in Chapter 12 to make sure they are on your plan and make a list and don't fray from it.

> ➢ 3 proteins (examples: extra-lean ground beef, skinless chicken breast, salmon)
> ➢ 3 vegetables (examples: fresh green beans, frozen broccoli, Romaine lettuce)
> ➢ 3 fruits (examples: apples, grapefruits, frozen blueberries)
> ➢ 3 grains (examples: Old Fashioned oatmeal, wild rice, sweet potatoes)
> ➢ 3 fats (examples: flaxseed oil, walnuts, avocados)

Now what are you going to do when you get home from the grocery store with all this fresh and healthy food? First, you're going to put it away. Most everything is perishable so it will either have to go into the refrigerator or freezer. Certain oils don't have to be refrigerated such as extra virgin olive oil and coconut oil, but make sure you read your food labels as you don't want your new foods to go rancid. Most grains and nuts also do not have to be refrigerated.

You are now ready for a great week of healthy meals. Remember to balance all your meals with protein, carbohydrates, and fats. You may refer back to Chapter 5 (Don't Make Healthy Eating a Chore) to review the 9 principles of healthy eating. If you are a very busy person who doesn't have time to cook, then you may want to prepare some of your foods ahead of time. Carve out a couple of hours one day of the week. Weekends are best for most people to do both their grocery shopping and food preparations. Cook all your meats and store them in the refrigerator for the week. Then you can pull what you want when you're ready to eat and just reheat. Having the meat already cooked also helps to prepare other dishes quickly when you get home from work. In lieu of reheating, meats can be sliced and made into stir-fry, stews, and chili dishes quickly and easily. Vegetables can be chopped and stored in separate containers or baggies. Some may even be cooked ahead of time for busy people, or frozen can be bought and cooked in the microwave with a little water in just four to seven minutes. Oats and rice can be prepared ahead of time and even frozen. Just take out what you need when you need it and reheat with a tablespoon of water.

Planning and preparing foods doesn't have to be a chore. You may find some delicious recipes in the next chapter that are extremely simple to prep and cook. Don't be intimidated. For what you can whip up in the kitchen for a meal saves you that much more time in the drive-thru lane at a fast food restaurant. You'll be much healthier and happier!

Meal Planning Steps for Phase 2 & 3 Users

You are a planner! Staying organized and sticking to the plan is your goal. Following are five steps to help you plan for healthy meals.

1. **Pick a day for meal planning.** Pick a day out of your week to do your planning and food prepping and schedule those days on your calendar. You will need about three hours to write your meal plan, do your grocery shopping, and prepare some of your foods for the upcoming week. You may need less time in future weeks as you may want to rotate your menu plans that you've already created. Save your grocery lists for those plans as well. (You may find planning forms in the appendix.)

2. **Plan your meals.** On your scheduled days, you are going to plan all your meals from breakfast to bedtime snack for seven days of the week. Every single meal does not have to be different. People are creatures of habit and you may be this way as well. You may find that there are only two or three different breakfast meals you like, so you will most likely eat those meals twice per week. Most people rotate between three breakfasts, six lunches, and nine dinners. Your ratio may even be smaller. After you have planned for a week or two, you may find that you are done planning meals for a while and just rotate those that you've already created. Once you have these down, the next planning session is faster and easier.

3. **Make your grocery lists.** After your meal plans are complete, add up each of your foods for the week and make your grocery list.

SIMPLE = EASY!

4. **Prepping your foods.** Once the groceries are home and put away, you can start prepping and cooking some of your foods to make it easier throughout the week. Following are some things you can do to be prepared for the week.

   - Season, marinade, and cook all your meats. Grilling is the easiest and fastest way to cook a large amount and saves times for the rest of the week. However, if you do have time to cook each day, you can still season, marinade, and store in your refrigerator or freezer for the allotted meal times.

- Chop your vegetables and put each into separate containers or bags within the refrigerator.
- Cook starchy carbs (i.e., oats and rice) and store in the refrigerator.
- Portion out foods like cottage cheese, Greek yogurt, and protein powder and put into small containers in the refrigerator or pantry.
- Bag servings of nuts (i.e., walnuts, almonds, pecans, etc.) to add to your cottage cheese, Greek yogurt, and protein pudding snacks.
- Pack lunches and snacks for work.

You will find that planning and preparation will help you throughout each day. You won't feel so bombarded with the thought of meals, and you will have so much more time for the other things life brings you. Besides, you will have the feeling of accomplishment that you stayed on track. By staying on course, you even receive a BONUS → fat loss, body transformation, and good health!

Invest in Useful Kitchen Utensils

Cooking doesn't have to be difficult. You don't need a bunch of fancy equipment to make tasty and healthy meals. Just invest in kitchen utensils and appliances you know you will use. Below are some suggestions, though the list may include equipment that Phase 1 and 2 users may not need. Most likely, you will have the majority of these already.

- ➢ Digital kitchen scale that can measure ounces and grams.
- ➢ Measuring cups and measuring spoons.
- ➢ Mixing spoons, spatulas, vegetable peeler, garlic press, and scissors.
- ➢ Can opener and strainer.
- ➢ Chopping, cutting, and steak knives.
- ➢ Food processor, blender, or smoothie machine.
- ➢ Toaster oven (the kind that comes with rotisserie capability is nice).
- ➢ Stove top or electric skillet.
- ➢ Gas or charcoal grill.
- ➢ Broiler pan.
- ➢ Baking dishes.
- ➢ Canning jars (for homemade salsas, dressings, marinades, and rubs).
- ➢ Sealable bags (for storing portioned meats or other foods).
- ➢ Mixing bowls.
- ➢ Microwavable containers with lids.

14 – Simple Recipes and Ideas

What you will learn in this section:
- ✓ How to prepare simple recipes.
- ✓ Tips for vegetables.
- ✓ Tips for leftovers.

Remember that food preparation and cooking doesn't need to be gourmet and difficult with a ton of ingredients. For success, it must be simple! The following pages will give you some ideas and recipes for a variety of foods to prepare throughout the day. In fact, you may also use most of these recipes to prepare for several days of food, especially if you are working and don't have much time to cook throughout the week. Following are the types of food that you will find recipes and tips for that will be included in this chapter:

- ➢ Proteins (i.e., lean meats, poultry, pork tenderloin, fish, and seafood)
- ➢ Marinades
- ➢ Rubs
- ➢ Vegetable tips for fresh and frozen
- ➢ Vegetable salads
- ➢ Salsas
- ➢ Salad dressings
- ➢ Snacks

Protein Recipes and Ideas

If you recall from Chapter 5, proteins are very important nutritional building blocks. Your body composition depends on protein. Following are a few recipes and ideas to help you prepare and cook as simply as possible. Marinades and rubs add great flavoring to your meats, and recipes can be found on pages 214-215. Most of these recipes will make more than one serving. For most, you can prepare enough for your entire family for dinner. If you are the only one to prepare for, then you will have a few leftovers which only need to be reheated. This saves you time!

Lean Red Meat

➤ **Flank Steaks**. Marinade and let sit overnight or at least for 30-60 minutes, and grill on each side for 5 minutes.
➤ **Filet Mignon**. Rub and let sit for 20-30 minutes; grill for 5 minutes on each side.
➤ **Chuck Steak Kabobs**. Marinade and let sit overnight or at least for 30-60 minutes. Place on skewers with veggies of your choice. Grill for 5 minutes on each side.
➤ **Burgers**. Add an egg, chopped onions, minced garlic, and a little sea salt and black pepper. Form into patties and grill for 5 minutes on each side. Top with salsa.

Chicken Breast

➤ **Skillet Chicken**. Thinly slice chicken breast where it is only about ¼" thick. Sprinkle with rub and cook in skillet with a little EVOO (extra virgin olive oil) for 4-5 minutes on each side.
➤ **Baked Chicken**. Place chicken breast in a 9x13 glass casserole dish, and pour low-sodium chicken broth over chicken. Bake at 350 degrees Fahrenheit for about 25-30 minutes (or until done).
➤ **Grilled Chicken**. Marinade for 20-30 minutes and grill.
➤ **Chicken Stir-Fry**. Slice chicken breast into thin bite-sized pieces. Stir-fry in electric skillet with veggies of choice and a little coconut oil. While cooking, add a little tamari sauce, sea salt, and black pepper.

Turkey

- **Crockpot Turkey Breast**. Remove giblets from turkey breast (with bone). Rinse well and put whole turkey breast into large crockpot. Cover with water, add pinch of sea salt, pepper, and spices of your choice. Cook all day on low (about 8 hours).
- **Turkey Meatballs**. Mix 2.5 pounds lean ground turkey with 1 egg, ½ medium chopped onion, 2 garlic cloves, 1 tsp. dried basil, 1 tsp. sea salt, and pinch of black pepper. Roll into balls and broil approximately 4-5 minutes on each side.

Pork

- **Grilled Pork Tenderloin**. Slice tenderloin into ¾" thick pieces. Sprinkle with rub on both sides and let sit for 30-60 minutes. Grill for 5 minutes on each side.
- **Pork Stir-Fry**. Cut tenderloin into very thin slices. Marinade overnight or at least for 30-60 minutes. Stir-fry in electric skillet with veggies of choice and a little EVOO (extra virgin olive oil) or coconut oil.

Fish

- **Baked Salmon**. Marinade salmon flanks with a mix of ¼ cup Tamari sauce, 1 garlic clove, and pinch of sea salt and black pepper. Bake on 400 degrees Fahrenheit for approx. 20 minutes.
- **Fried Tilapia**. First, dip tilapia fillets in almond milk. Second, dip fillets in a mixture of ground nuts or flour (almonds or walnuts), as well as a pinch of sea salt and black pepper. Make sure skillet is very hot. Then turn to medium-high and cook fish in coconut oil for 4 minutes on each side.

HELPFUL TIP!
Include protein in every single meal and snack!
Protein is thermogenic and leads to increased metabolism.
A faster metabolism = more body fat burned!

Shrimp

- **Buttered Shrimp & Scallops**. Heat butter in skillet. Add shrimp and scallops and cook for about 5 minutes (shrimp should be pink, not gray).
- **Coconut Shrimp**. Roll shrimp in beaten egg and then unsweetened coconut. Heat coconut oil in large skillet until hot. Add shrimp. Cook for about 2 minutes on each side (should be fried golden when done).
- **Steamed Shrimp**. Buy pre-steamed at butcher/fish counter at your supermarket!

Crab

- **Coconut Crab Cakes**. Mix together 2 eggs, 2 Tbs. EVOO mayonnaise, 2 tsp. Worcestershire sauce, 1 tsp. lemon juice, 1 Tbs. dry mustard, 1 tsp. Old Bay seasoning, 1 tsp. dried parsley, and ½ cup unsweetened coconut. Fold in 16 oz. claw crab meat. Make into patties and fry in skillet with coconut oil for about 4 minutes on each side.
- **Steamed Crabs**. Buy pre-steamed at butcher/fish counter at your supermarket!

Canned Tuna

- **Tuna & Egg Salad**. Drain 6 oz. tuna (in water) and place in bowl. Add 2 chopped hard-boiled eggs, 3 Tbs. chopped red onion, 4 Tbs. EVOO mayonnaise, 1 tsp. celery seed or salt, and 1 Tbs. dry mustard. Mix well. Serve on Romaine lettuce.
- **Easy Tuna Cakes**. Drain 12 oz. Albacore tuna and mix with 2 whole eggs, 2 Tbs. EVOO mayonnaise, 1 tsp. Worcestershire sauce, 1 minced garlic clove, ⅓ cup ground oats, and 2 tsp. Old Bay. Make patties. Cook in heated skillet with EVOO for 4 minutes on each side.

Canned Salmon

> **Easy Salmon Patties**. Drain one 14.75 oz. can of salmon (red sockeye is nutritionally the best). Mix in bowl with 2 eggs, 1 small chopped onion, 1 tsp. parsley, and 1 tsp. black pepper. Make into patties and cook in heated (hot) skillet with coconut oil for 4 minutes on each side.

> **Salmon Stir-Fry**. Drain one 14.75 oz. can of salmon (or fresh). Heat skillet and add a little EVOO. Throw in veggies of choice, salmon, minced garlic, 2-3 Tbs. Tamari sauce. Cook until veggies are tender.

Egg Whites

> **Spinach Egg White Quiche**. Mix 12 egg whites, ¼ cup fat-free milk, one 10 oz. frozen spinach (de-thawed & drained), 1-½ cup shredded Monterey Jack cheese, ½ tsp. black pepper, and ½ tsp. dry mustard. Pour into quiche or deep pie dish (sprayed with EVOO oil), and bake on 350 degrees Fahrenheit for 40 minutes on or until center sets.

> **Egg White & Avocado Salad**. Mix 6 hard-boiled egg whites (chopped), 1 chopped avocado, 1 chopped celery stalk, 1 small chopped Granny Smith apple, 2 Tbs. EVOO mayonnaise, 2 tsp. lemon juice, ½ tsp. sea salt, and ¼ tsp. black pepper. Serve topped over butter lettuce.

Protein Powder

> **Protein Oatmeal Waffles**. Mix 1-½ scoops vanilla protein powder, ½ cup ground oatmeal, and 4 egg whites. Spray hot waffle iron with butter spray, and pour batter into waffle and cook as waffle maker instructs. Top waffles with fruit, walnuts, and sugar-free syrup made with Splenda.

> **Banana Pancakes**. Mix 1 scoop vanilla protein powder, 1 Tbs. psyllium powder, ¼ cup almond milk, and ½ mashed banana. Pour batter into hot skillet and cook until holes form in the top. Then flip and cook for 1 minute more. Top pancakes with fruit and pecans if desired, as well as sugar-free syrup made with Splenda.

Marinades and Rubs to Make Yummy Meats

Healthy foods don't need to be boring! In fact, they can actually feel sinful with the right marinades and rubs. Following are a few marinades that can be made and stored with air-tight jars in the refrigerator. Meat rubs can be stored in air-tight containers in your pantry and used as needed. Prepation time is minimal at five minutes.

Steak Marinade	Poultry Marinade	Pork Tenderloin Marinade
•½ cup EVOO	•¼ cup water	•¼ cup EVOO
•¼ cup Tamari sauce	•¼ cup Tamari sauce	•¼ cup Tamari sauce
•2-½ Tbs. red wine vinegar	•1 tsp. sweet red chili pepper sauce (optional)	•3 Tbs. dijon honey mustard
•2 Tbs. lemon juice	•¾ tsp. lemon juice	•1 clove garlic, minced
•1 TBS. dijon mustard	•¼ cup Stevia in the Raw or granulated Splenda	•sea salt, pinch
•½ onion, finely chopped or minced	•¼ tsp. onion powder	•black pepper, pinch
•1 garlic clove, minced	•¼ tsp. ground ginger	•This marinade recipe is good for about a 2 pound tenderloin.
•1-½ Tbs. ground black pepper		

HELPFUL TIP!
Marinade meats either overnight or for a few hours for best taste. This allows the flavors to soak into the meats.

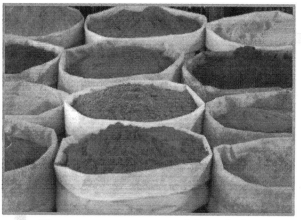

Flavor your meats with rubs!

Flavor your meats with rubs made of spices and herbs as they have more disease-fighting antioxidants than most vegetables and fruits. You may prepare the following rubs, store, and use as needed.

Barbecue Rub

¼ cup paprika

¼ cup Stevia in the raw or granulated Splenda

1-⅓ Tbs. dry mustard

1-⅓ Tbs. onion powder

1-⅓ Tbs. garlic powder

1 Tbs. dried basil

2 tsp. ground bay leaves

½ Tbs. savory

½ Tbs. ground coriander

½ Tbs. dried thyme

½ Tbs. ground black pepper

½ Tbs. white pepper

¼ tsp. kosher salt

Essence Rub

3 Tbs. chili powder

2 Tbs. paprika

1 Tbs. cayenne

1 Tbs. ground cumin

1 Tbs. ground coriander

1 Tbs. kosher salt

1 Tbs. black pepper

1 Tbs. garlic powder

1 Tbs. onion powder

Fresh Veggie Tips and Recipes

Below are some tips for fresh vegetable preparation. Choose vegetables that satisfy your palette. If you don't know of any that you like, experiment as there are literally hundreds to choose from. Vegetable items can be chopped or sliced and stored in airtight containers in the refrigerator for easy access to meals throughout the week. They can be eaten raw, cooked in stir fry, grilled on skewers, steamed, or made into salads.

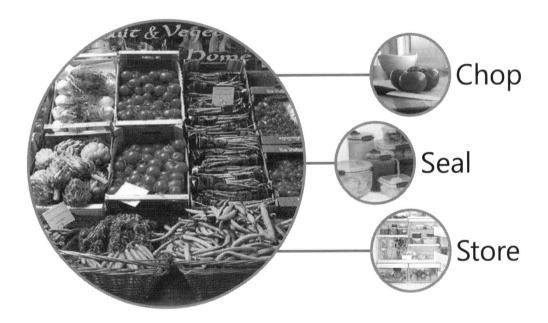

Frozen Veggie Tips!

Frozen veggies can be just as healthy as fresh. Buy without preservatives and sauces. Birds Eye Steam Fresh and family packs are easy to prepare. Just put in microwavable dish with a few tablespoons of water, and cook on high 4 to 7 minutes.

Cucumber, Tomato & Onion Salad

Mix all ingredients. Chill before serving, or let stand for at least 10 minutes.

- large cucumbers, peeled & thinly sliced
- 1 pint cherry or grape tomatoes, halved
- ½ medium sweet onion, sliced
- 2 Tbs. fresh chopped -or- 1 Tbs. dried parsley
- 1 Tbs. apple cider vinegar
- 1 Tbs. EVOO
- sea salt and black pepper to taste
- Mix all ingredients. Let stand for 10 minutes.

Carrot & Apple Salad

Blend all ingredients together until smooth. Chill before serving.

- ½ pound carrots, peeled and grated
- 1 Granny Smith apple, peeled and chopped
- ¼ cup apple cider vinegar
- ½ cup EVOO
- 2 Tbs. water
- 1 tsp. poppy seeds
- kosher salt, pinch

Broccoli Salad

Blend all ingredients and allow to chill before serving.

- 1 head fresh broccoli, chopped into bite-size
- ½ medium red onion, finely chopped
- ¼ cup golden raisins
- ⅓ cup slivered almonds
- ½ cup EVOO mayonnaise
- ¼ cup Stevia in the Raw or granulated Splenda

Fresh Salsa Recipes

Salsas are great toppings for meats, fish, and even steamed vegetables. It can be stored in airtight containers in the refrigerator and is usually good for about three to four days. Preparation time is five to 10 minutes, depending on how fast you can chop.

Homemade Salsa

Mix and chill for 30 minutes before serving.

- 3 large ripe tomatoes (remove seeds), chopped
- ¼ cup finely chopped sweet onion
- 1 large hot chili pepper (jalapeno or Serrano)
- 2 small cloves minced garlic
- 2-3 TBS fresh chopped cilantro
- 1-½ Tbs. lime juice
- sea salt and pepper to taste

Fresh Mango Salsa

Mix and chill for 30 minutes before serving.

- 1 mango, diced
- ½ each red & green peppers, diced
- ¼ cup green onions, thinly sliced
- 1 clove minced garlic
- 1 Tbs. EVOO
- 1 Tbs. balsamic vinegar
- 1 tsp. Stevia in the Raw -or- granulated Splenda

> **HELPFUL TIP!**
> *Salsas are nutritious and a great way to flavor your meats, starches, and veggies! Prepare them ahead of time as they will keep for 3-4 days.*

Salad Dressing Recipes

What's a salad without a bit of dressing? Make your own as it will be fresh and free of preservatives and sugars. For each recipe, combine all ingredients and whisk well. Put in airtight jar and store in refrigerator. If you prefer to use fresh herbs, the dried teaspoon equivalent is one tablespoon for fresh. Preparation time is five minutes.

Creamy Tarragon

- ½ cup EVOO
- 2 TBS. tarragon vinegar
- 2 TBS. dijon mustard
- 1 tsp. dried tarragon
- ½ tsp. sea salt
- 1/8 tsp. white pepper
- 1 tsp. Stevia in the Raw -or- granulated Splenda

Balsamic Vinaigrette

- ¾ cup EVOO
- ¼ cup balsamic vinegar
- 1 TBS. dijon mustard
- ½ tsp. dried marjarom or oregano
- ½ tsp. dried basil

Garlic Herb Vinaigrette

- 1-½ cup EVOO
- ½ cup apple cider vinegar
- 1 TBS. dijon mustard
- 3 small cloves minced garlic
- 1 tsp. dried oregano
- 1 tsp. dried thyme
- pinch of sea salt & pepper

Flaxseed Tarragon

- ½ cup flaxseed oil
- ¼ cup tarragon vinegar
- 1 clove minced garlic
- 1 tsp. dried tarragon
- ½ tsp. dried parsley
- ½ tsp. chives

Quick and Easy Snack Recipes and Ideas

Nutrition balance should be included in all of your meals, including snacks. Below are quick and easy snack recipes and ideas.

Cottage Cheese

- **Idea 1**. Low-fat cottage cheese mixed with blueberries and walnuts
- **Idea 2**. Low-fat cottage cheese mixed with cucumber slices and chia seeds
- **Idea 3**. Low-fat cottage cheese mixed with low-carb vanilla protein powder, strawberry slices, and almond slivers
- **Idea 4**. Low-fat cottage cheese mixed with cocoa power, blueberries, and natural peanut butter

Greek Yogurt

- **Idea 1**. Plain Greek yogurt mixed with pineapple chunks and almond butter
- **Idea 2**. Plain Greek yogurt mixed with chocolate protein powder, natural peanut butter, and raspberries
- **Idea 3**. Plain Greek yogurt mixed with pure pumpkin puree and pecans
- **Idea 4**. Plain Greek yogurt mixed with cocoa powder, blueberries, and flaxseed

HELPFUL TIP!

Most people with lactose intolerance can handle cottage cheese and Greek yogurt. However, you may find that they are not for you. That's okay as there are plenty of other foods you can try.

Hard-boiled Eggs

- ➤ **Idea 1**. Hard-boiled eggs with carrot and celery sticks
- ➤ **Idea 2**. Hard-boiled egg salad made with chopped carrots, bell peppers, and EVOO mayonnaise
- ➤ **Idea 3**. Hard-boiled eggs with grapefruit
- ➤ **Idea 4**. Hard-boiled eggs mixed with canned tuna in water (drained), chopped onions and celery, mustard, and EVOO mayonnaise

Natural Deli Meats

- ➤ **Idea 1**. Natural turkey slices rolled with natural cheese and green bell pepper slices
- ➤ **Idea 2**. Natural chicken breast slices rolled with red bell pepper slices and avocado
- ➤ **Idea 3**. Natural lean roast beef slices rolled with Swiss cheese, green onions, and sun-dried tomatoes
- ➤ **Idea 4**. Butter lettuce wrapped with natural lean roast beef, red bell pepper slices, and avocado

HELPFUL TIP!

Balanced snacks are just as important as balanced meals. Getting a source of protein, carbohydrate, and fat will provide you with necessary nutrients, boost your immune system, and burn body fat.

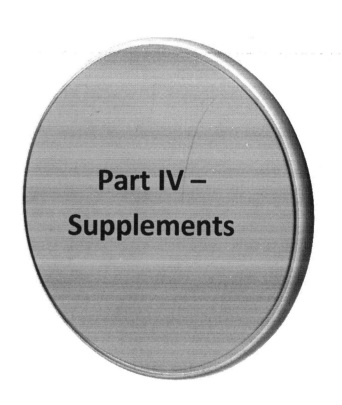

Part IV –
Supplements

15 – Supplements are Insurance

What you will learn in this section:
- ✓ Which supplements should be used as your body's insurance.
- ✓ What supplements are helpful for special needs.

With the health and fitness industry being driven by supplements, most people are prone to curiosity about them. Be careful! You will find tons of advertisements via television, radio, billboards, and magazines claiming that a particular supplement will help you lose body fat or provide some "magical" solution to your needs. Most of these advertisements are hype, and most of these supplements are expensive filler pills. Fillers are usually binders that hold the effective ingredient (i.e., vitamin, mineral, or other nutrient) together in a form that you can swallow. Fillers may include sugar, salt, yeast, wheat, gluten, soy, milk, egg, fish, shellfish, nut, and preservatives. Though some of these ingredients may not harm your health, there are some supplements filled with toxic and harmful ingredients such as aspartame and coal tar. Medical professionals even warn patients about trans or hydrogenated fats because they are linked to high cholesterol and heart disease, yet many supplements are filled with hydrogenated soybean oil. Artificial flavoring or coloring may also be added to supplements to make them appealing to the consumer. Many gel caps even contain animal products from pig and cow which dismay vegetarians and vegans.

Determining if a Supplement Works

How do you know if a particular supplement is good or hype? The truth is by trial and error. If you find a supplement that works, then keep it. If it doesn't work, throw it out. Supplements may also work for one person but not another. The best way to determine if a supplement is working is by trying one at a time. Some supplements claim that you will get results with the day that you take them (such as ibuprofen for pain). Others may need to be built upon for several weeks before results are seen. Read your labels or Google the supplement on the internet to find what you should expect.

Five Staple Supplements[126]

All supplements are an option, but staple supplements will provide your body with insurance. When your intake of certain vitamins, minerals, or phytonutrients is low via food, staple supplements will fill in the gap. Below are five supplements recommended as staples to your nutrition plan.

1. **Protein powder.** Use a high quality isolate milk protein blend as it is the purest of protein powders. Egg and rice protein blends are fine too if you cannot tolerate dairy products; however, isolate milk proteins usually have little if any lactose and most with intolerances can handle this form of protein. Protein supplement's food equivalent is a protein source food such as lean beef, poultry, pork tenderloin, fish, egg whites, and dairy products. If you are getting adequate amounts of whole food protein sources, your use of protein powder supplementation will be infrequent. You may use this supplementation when you don't have whole food protein sources available. Most will blend with water, and you can take it on the go.

2. **Multi-vitamin/Multi-mineral.** A good quality multi-vitamin/multi-mineral supplement should be taken every day, unless you are very conscientious about your diet as well as making it varied. Take this supplement with food, especially when your diet is lacking.

3. **Fish oil.** A fish oil supplement high in Omega-3 content should contain at least 30 percent EPA and DHA. You may also get fish oil from whole food sources like cold water fish (i.e., salmon, mackerel, halibut, sardines, tuna, and herring). Daily recommended dose of fish oil is two to three grams total of Omega-3 rich fish oil.

4. **Greens/Berry Powder.** A greens/berry powder (or pill form) supplement is rich in vitamins and minerals, high in anti-oxidants, and strongly alkaline. Take this supplement when your intake of vegetables and fruits is less than 10 servings per day. (This supplement does not count as a vegetable or fruit block in meal planning.)

5. **Branched-chain amino acids (BCAAs).** Though you will be naturally taking in BCAAs through a protein-rich nutrition plan, BCAAs should be taken during all strenuous or high-intensity workouts, especially during body fat loss phases. This will help to preserve muscle tissue. Take BCAAs in powder or pill form before, during, or after exercise. The supplemental range for BCAAs should range from 1.5 to 6 grams for leucine and 800 mg. to 3 grams for both isoleucine and valine. When shopping for BCAAs, look for one with vitamin B6 (pyridoxine) and glutamic acid.[127]

Supplements to Curb Cravings

- **r-Alpha lipoic acid.** For those with poor carbohydrate tolerance, use r-Alpha lipoic acid to improve insulin sensitivity and reduce insulin response. This supplement is also good for those who are working on weight loss goals. Recommended dosage is 100 mg. three times per day. [128]

- **Chromium.** Include 200 to 600 micrograms daily (can be divided doses) to lower blood glucose (sugar) levels. Because chromium helps to breakdown proteins, carbohydrates, and fats into energy, it is a good supplement for those working on fat loss goals.[129]

Supplements to Stimulate Metabolism[130]

- **Green tea extract.** Include 400 mg. of green tea extract one to two times per day to stimulate metabolism while working on body fat loss goals. Be sure your green tea extract has the most active component called EGCG (epigallocatechin gallate).

- **Conjugated linoleic acid (CLA).** During weight loss phases, take 2.5 to five grams of CLA daily in either a single or divided dose. CLA stimulates the metabolism, causes fat cells to die, and down-regulates leptin.

Supplements to Support Training[131]

- **Beta alanine.** During high lactate activity, take 1,000 mg. three times per day. This supplement may cause tingling or flushing of the skin but is not harmful.

- **Creatine.** To help supply energy to all cells of the body, especially the muscles, take five grams once per day.

- **Tyrosine and phosphatidylcholine.** During high-volume training phases, take 2,000 to 3,000 mg. of tyrosine with 1,000 mg. of choline (not to be exceeded) after exercise. Tyrosine and phosphatidylcholine helps reduce central nervous system fatigue.

Supplements to Improve Sleep During Intense Training[132]

- **Valerian root.** Take 400 mg. approximately one hour before bedtime to improve sleep quality during high intensity training and energy deficit menu plans. Choose the extract form over the dried root.

- **Phosphatidylserine.** Take 300 mg. at dinner and 300 mg. one hour before bedtime to improve sleep quality during high-stress periods. Take with food.

- **Melatonin.** Take 3 mg. 30 minutes before bedtime to help you fall asleep. Melatonin is a natural hormone that helps control your sleep and wake cycles.[133]

Note: Use only one sleep supplement – not all three mentioned above.

Your Dreams (Afterword)

> **"Fearlessness is the gateway to success.**
> **One should shun all kinds of fear." ~Riq Veda**

You have a dream. You desire a beautiful and healthy body. Many of us have dreams, but the thing that usually holds us back from obtaining those dreams is *fear*. It doesn't have to be so! In your hands is the very tool to help you conquer everything you ever hoped for. It is your gateway to the rest of your life.

We have all imagined our futures. I'm sure you've imagined yourself as that beautiful slim and fit model on the cover of Oxygen Magazine. If you're a guy, you may have imagined yourself as the buff bodybuilder type. Maybe your imagination doesn't include so much vanity. Instead, you've imagined just being able to get down on the floor to play with your kids without feeling like you can't get back up. Or, you've thought about playing baseball or dodge ball with them without being out of breath. Maybe you would just like good health and vitality. Have you ever thought about your elder years? What would they be like? Would you be one of the folks we see in our local community rolling around on a motorized chair because they can't actually walk due to their weight and health? Or, have you imagined that you will be the super hero grandparent that can still run with the young ones? We can all be super heroes of our lives if we only treat our bodies with a bit of compassion and love.

Recall my quote in my introduction, "Food can be used as a poison or a prescription. Why not use it as a prescription for good health?" Our bodies rely on the right nutrients for health. They feed every single cell within our bodies so that they can do all the wonderful things you've imagined for your life. Maybe you feel like you've done too much damage to your body to ever recover and fulfill your dreams. That's when you need to get rid of that stinkin' thinking. Remember I was only given five years to live after being diagnosed with cancer. That was over 19 years ago! I have also conquered other major health issues that were supposed to debilitate me for the rest of my life. I never gave up, and you don't have to either. Our miracle to a healthy weight and life surrounds us. It's not in the latest fad pill or diet, and it's not in conventional medicine. It's in nature – *living* foods!

The information I have provided you is nothing new, but it seems to have been kept a secret for the last several decades. Why? Unfortunately, people get bored and are always looking for something new to try. Not only that! We also live in a hustle bustle society where we want *quick and easy*. Therefore, businesses have only touched on what we have desired without realizing the actual consequences of using their products. Now it's time to go back to the old in which we have forgotten. That is eating *real* foods that are actually made for our bodies. *One Size Does NOT Fit All Diet Plan* takes you back to the roots of good nutrition. It teaches you what types of food feed your body to help it function well. Not only that, it teaches you how to time your foods so that your body can function optimally. Models and athletes have utilized these same principles for years. As you can see, it works! Not only will it work for them, but it will work for YOU as well.

I understand that breaking old habits is difficult. However, I know that you can do it! If it takes a month of working hard on replacing one old habit with one new, it's worth it. You are worth it! Remember → no more fears! Take this plan one step at a time, and you will succeed. It's only the first step to living the life you've dreamed of.

Blessings!

P.S. As you embark on this wonderful journey to health and happiness, please promise me one thing. Contact me after you have made some progress. I would love to see before and after photos, as well as hear about your journey. You may contact me at Abby@911BodyResQ.com or on Facebook at https://www.facebook.com/Abby.911BodyResQ. I promise you I won't bite.

P.S.S. I have one last request. As you know, my only goal is to help anyone seeking weight loss and health success. If I've helped you in any way, would you please leave a review for my book on Amazon.com?

Share the Wealth!

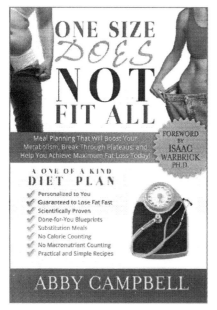

Why not share this book with your family and friends? It's the perfect gift, especially for anyone who may be struggling with healthy habits, dieting, and weight loss. As my gift to you, I am offering a substantial discount with FREE shipping. Please see the discount schedule below for *One Size Does NOT Fit All Diet Plan* which retails for $19.95.

I am only able to provide these generous discounts on a non-refundable basis when payment accompanies your order. You may make payment by charging the books to your credit card (i.e., Visa, MasterCard, American Express), by personal or company check, or through PayPal. In fact, all payments go through the PayPal merchant system, but you do not need a PayPal account to make payment. Go to www.AbbyCampbellOnline.com to purchase. Books will be shipped within 24 business hours.

Customer Appreciation Discount Schedule for Quantity Purchases		
2-4 copies	20% discount	$15.96 each
5-49 copies	30% discount	$13.97 each
50-99 copies	40% discount	$11.97 each
100+ copies	50% discount	$9.98 each

Appendix A: Self-Evaluation Form

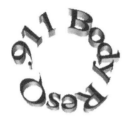

Self-Evaluation

List five current behaviors that are preventing you from achieving your goals. Next to each current behavior, write a new behavior that will allow you to achieve your goals.

	Current Behavior	New Behavior
1		
2		
3		
4		
5		

You may go to http://AbbyCampbellOnline.com to print blank forms.

Appendix B: Goals Planned Form

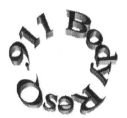

Goals Planned

What are your top five fat loss, fitness, and health goals? Also, list two actions you can do immediately to move towards achieving those goals.

	Goal Description	Action #1	Action #2
1			
2			
3			
4			
5			

You may go to http://AbbyCampbellOnline.com to print blank forms.

Appendix C: Goal Deadlines Form

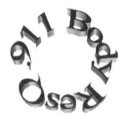

Goal Deadlines

List your deadline dates for your top five fat loss, fitness, and health goals. Also, list your overall deadline for all goals.

	Goal Description	Deadline Date	
1			
2			**Overall Deadline Date**
3			
4			
5			

You may go to http://AbbyCampbellOnline.com to print blank forms.

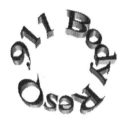

Value of Goals

What is the cost of achieving your goals?	What is the cost of NOT achieving your goals?
What will you experience if you succeed in your goals?	**What will you NOT experience if you do NOT succeed in your goals?**

You may go to http://AbbyCampbellOnline.com to print blank forms.

Appendix E: Weight Measurements Form

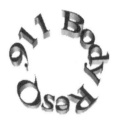

Weight Measurements

Date	Weight		Date	Weight		Date	Weight

NOTE: For consistency, weigh yourself at the same time each week, preferably in the morning after awaking and using the restroom.

You may go to http://AbbyCampbellOnline.com to print blank forms.

Appendix F: Girth Measurements Form

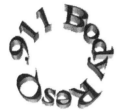

Girth Measurements

Body Parts	Dates				
Neck (base)					
Shoulders (widest)					
Bicep (left)					
Chest (nipple line)					
Waist (narrowest)					
Hips (widest front view)					
Thigh (Left midpoint)					
Calf (left widest)					

NOTE: For better accuracy, use a myotape by AccuFitness to ensure results are correct (may be obtained through Amazon.com). Also, measure each body part at the same exact position. Thighs are the most difficult to measure accurately. A helpful tip is to write down the number of inches above the mid knee cap at first measurement. Use this number with future measurements. Also for consistency, measure yourself at the same time each week, preferably in the morning after awaking and using the restroom.

You may go to http://AbbyCampbellOnline.com to print blank forms.

Appendix G: Caliper Measurements Form

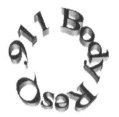

Caliper Measurements

Skinfold Sites	Dates				
Chest					
Abdominal					
Thigh					
Tricep					
Subscapular					
Suprailiac					
Midaxillary					

NOTE: For best accuracy, please have the same person take skinfold measurements (preferably a qualified personal trainer).

You may go to http://AbbyCampbellOnline.com to print blank forms.

Appendix H: Monthly Pictures Form

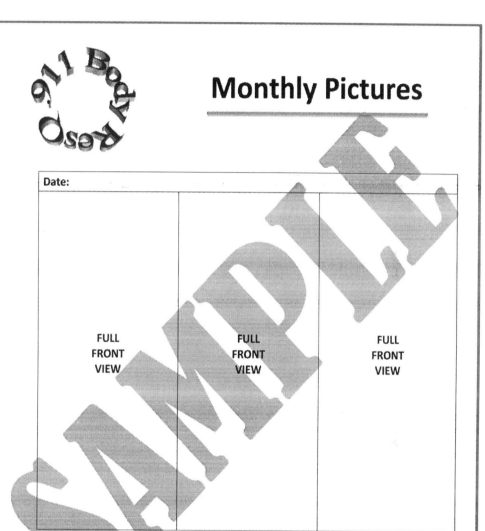

Monthly Pictures

911 Body ReSO

Date:

FULL FRONT VIEW	FULL FRONT VIEW	FULL FRONT VIEW

NOTE: Take pictures monthly with your girth measurements, preferably in the morning after awakening and using the bathroom.

You may go to http://AbbyCampbellOnline.com to print blank forms.

Appendix I: Phase 2 Meal Planning Worksheet – Rest Days

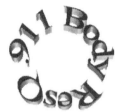

Phase 2 Nutrition Planning:
Daily Meal Planning Worksheet
Rest & Active Recovery Days

Meal	Protein	Veggie	Fat
Meal 1			
Meal 2			
Meal 3			
Meal 4			
Meal 5			
Meal 6			

NOTE: Please refer to Chapter 6 – Phase 2: Learn How to Build Your Healthy Plate when building your menus.

You may go to http://AbbyCampbellOnline.com to print blank forms.

Appendix L: Phase 3 Meal Planning Worksheet – Rest Days

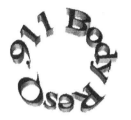

Phase 3 Nutrition Planning:
Daily Meal Planning Worksheet
Rest & Active Recovery Days

Calorie Plan: _____

Protein Blocks: _____   Veggie Blocks: _____   Fat Blocks: _____

Meal	Protein		Veggie		Fat
Meal 1					
Meal 2					
Meal 3					
Meal 4					
Meal 5					
Meal 6					
TOTAL					

You may go to http://AbbyCampbellOnline.com to print blank forms.

Appendix M: Phase 3 Meal Planning Worksheet – Normal Days

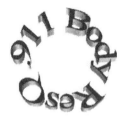

Phase 3 Nutrition Planning:
Daily Meal Planning Worksheet
Normal Workout & Cardio Days

Calorie Plan: _____   Protein Blocks: _____   Veggie Blocks: _____

Fruit Blocks: _____   Fat Blocks: _____

Meal	Protein	Veggie	Fruit	Fat
Meal 1				
Meal 2				
Meal 3				
Meal 4				
Meal 5				
Meal 6				
TOTAL				

You may go to http://AbbyCampbellOnline.com to print blank forms.

Appendix N: Phase 3 Meal Planning Worksheet – Strenuous Days

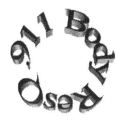

Phase 3 Nutrition Planning:
Daily Meal Planning Worksheet
Strenuous Workout Days

Calorie Plan: _____   Protein Blocks: _____   Veggie Blocks: _____

Fruit Blocks: _____   Starch Blocks: _____   Fat Blocks: _____

Meal	Protein	Veggie	Fruit	Starch	Fat
Meal 1					
Meal 2					
Meal 3					
Meal 4					
Meal 5					
Meal 6					
TOTAL					

You may go to http://AbbyCampbellOnline.com to print blank forms.

Recommended Reading

The following are books that you may not only enjoy, but you may be even more encouraged and motivated to living a healthy lifestyle.

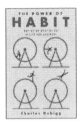 The Power of Habit: Why We Do What We Do in Life and Business (2012) by Charles Duhigg

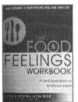 The Food and Feelings Workbook: A Full Course Meal on Emotional Health (2007) by Karen R. Koenig, LCSW, M.Ed.

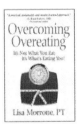 Overcoming Overeating: It's Not What You Eat, It's What's Eating You! (2007) by Lisa Morrone, PT

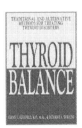 Thyroid Balance: Traditional and Alternative Methods for Treating Thyroid Disorder (2003) by Glenn S. Rothfield, MD, MA, and Deborah S. Romaine

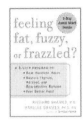 Feeling Fat, Fuzzy, or Frazzled? A 3-Step Program To Beat Hormone Havoc; Restore Thyroid, Adrenal, and Reproductive Balance; and Feel Better Fast! (2005) by Richard Shames, MD, and Karilee Shames, PhD, RN

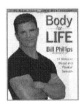 Body for Life: 12 Weeks to Mental and Physical Strength (1999) by Bill Phillips and Michael D'Orso

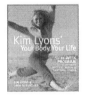 Your Body, Your Life: The 12-Week Program to Optimum Physical, Mental, and Emotional Fitness (2008) by Kim Lyons & Lara McGlashan.

Additional Resources

Carlson Labs
Providing only the highest quality nutritional supplements.
http://www.CarlsonLabs.com/

Eat Wild
Your source for finding safe, healthy, natural, and nutritious grass-fed beef, lamb, goats, bison, poultry, pork, dairy, and other wild edibles in your local area.
http://www.EatWild.com/

Food for Life
Certified organic ingredients and kosher. No genetically modified organisims, preservatives, shortenings, or refined sugars. Gluten and wheat free products (i.e., breads, pastas, and cereals) available. http://FoodForLife.com

Hampton Wellness Foundation
Promoting, engaging, and sustaining community health and wellness. Educating and empowering individuals and families on better lifestyle choices to prevent childhood and adult obesity. Transforming poor health and nutrition behaviors.
http://www.HamptonWellness.org

Local Harvest
Real food. Real farmers. Real community. Sign up for Community Supported Agriculture (CSA) by supporting your local, seasonal foods from your local farmer! http://www.localharvest.org/

New Life Path Fitness
New Life Path Fitness was founded of steering those on the wrong path of an unhappy sedentary lifestyle. The new path to a healthy, happy and active lifestyle has been laid down to endless rewards achieved through hard work and a no excuses attitude. http://www.NewLifePathFitness.com

NOW Foods
Providing value in products and services (supplements, personal care, sports nutrition, and food) that empower people to lead healthier lives.
http://www.NOWfoods.com/

Perfect Workout Calendar
Go ahead! Proudly display how committed you are! Stay on track with workouts! All calendars are dry erasable, and many include unique DVD holders for an up to a week's worth of workouts. Choose between 30, 60, and 90 day designs. Order your perfect workout calendar today!
http://www.PerfectWorkoutCalendar.com

Glossary

A

Addiction – a persistent and compulsive dependance on a substance (i.e., alcohol, drugs, and food).

Additive – a substance intentionally added to food during any stage to alter it, usually for taste or preservation.

Adrenal cortex – the outer layer of the adrenal gland that produces many steroid hormones, including cortisol, which regulates carbohydrate metabolism and the immune system while also maintaining blood pressure.

Adrenal gland – one of two endocrine glands located above each kidney and consists of a cortex (produces several steroid hormones) and a medulla (produces epinephrine).

Adrenaline – a hormone produced by the center part of the adrenal gland that responds to stress while increasing heart and pulse rates, blood pressure, as well as glucose and lipids.

Amino acids – organic compounds made by protein that the human body uses to build and repair body tissue.

Anabolic process – a metabolic process that uses cellular energy to construct larger molecules from smaller molecules.

Anabolism – metabolism's phase when simple substances are converted into more complex compounds of living tissue.

Antioxidants – a chemical compound that protects the body's cells from damaging effects of deterioration (free radicals).

B

Balanced diet – a diet that provides balance with all food groups (i.e., protein, carbohydrate, and fat).

Biochemical process – all the processes that involve chemical reactions in living organisms.

Blood sugar – the concentration of glucose in the blood.

Body composition – the relative between lean body mass proportions (i.e., bone, water, muscle, and vital organs) and fat mass (i.e., adipose tissue and intro-tissue fat deposits).

Body fats – the percentage of a person's body that is not composed of bone, water, muscle, and vital organs.

C

Calorie – a measure of energy expenditure equal to the amount of heat contained in foods and released by the body's oxidation.

Calorie/Carb Cycling – dietary pattern of cycling, or altering, calories and carbohydrates with high and low levels so that the body does not find homeostasis.

Carbohydrates – any of a group of organic compounds (i.e., sugars, starches, cellulose, and gums) that serves as a major energy source in the diet. One carbohydrate is equivalent to four calories.

Catabolism – metabolism's phase when complex compounds of living cells are broken down into more simple substances.

Cell – the simplest organism within the body that can have a life of its own; the body is dependent on all cell function as they work together to promote life.

Cortisol – a hormone produced by the outer portion of the adrenal gland when under stress and affects the metabolism of protein, glucose, and fats.

Cravings – a strong desire to consume a particular substance (i.e., alcohol, drugs, and food).

E

Energy – power that may be translated into motion, overcoming resistance, or causing a physical change.

Energy balance – a balanced relationship between all sources of energy intake (foods) and energy expenditure (exercise, daily activities, and vital function) and is usually evidenced by a steady body weight.

Energy deficit – an unbalanced relationship between all sources of energy intake (foods and energy) and energy expenditure (exercise, daily activities, and vital function) where energy intake is lower than energy expenditure and is usually evidenced by a a loss of body weight.

Energy density – a ratio of nutrient content to the total energy content. Energy dense foods provide few nutrients (i.e., vitamins, minerals, and phytonutrients) with a high level of calories.

Energy expenditure – the amount of energy used for exercise, daily activities, and vital function).

Energy intake – the amount of energy taken in from foods and beverages.

Estrogen – a group of steroid hormones that primarily regulate the growth, development, and function of the female reproductive system.

F

Fatigue – physical or mental weariness caused by excessive stimulation or prolonged exertion.

Fatty acids – dietary fat building blocks that are essential to the body for essential health.

Fiber – the part of vegetables, fruits, and grains that contain cellulose and are not digested by the body yet helps the intestines to absorb water which increases the bulk of stools and causes it to move more quickly through the colon.

Fluid balance – a balanced relationship between fluid intake and fluid expenditure.

Food binge – a period of uncontrolled and excessive indulgence in food and drink.

Food intolerance – an adverse reaction to food that does not involve the immune system.

Free radicals – high energy particles that richochet wildly and damage the body's cells.

G

Glucagon – a hormone produced by the pancreas to increase blood glucose levels.

Glucose – an essential component for energy production and is transported by blood and lymph to all the cells of the body where it is metabolized.

Gluten – a mixture of plant proteins occurring in grains such as wheat, barley, rye, and corn.

Glycemic index – a measure of the rate at which an ingested food causes glucose levels in the blood to rise.

Glycogen – a form of carbohydrate energy stored in the liver and muscle cells that can easily be converted into glucose to meet metabolic energy requirements.

Growth hormones – an anabolic hormone produced by the pituitary gland that promotes growth in bone, cartilage, and muscle.

H

Habits – a recurrent and usually unconscious pattern of behavior that is acquired through constant repetition.

Health – the general condition of body and mind which should be vigorous and free from disease.

Hormone – a chemical substance produced by an endocrine gland and transported by blood to a certain tissue in the body where it will exert a specific effect.

I

Imbalanced energy – an imbalanced relationship between all sources of energy intake (foods) and energy expenditure (exercise, daily activities, and vital function) and is usually evidenced by either weight loss or weight gain.

Inflammation – the reaction by the body to injury or infection and is characterized by swelling, heat, redness, or pain.

Insulin – a hormone released from the pancreas and is necessary for the metabolism of nutrients, including the regulation of blood sugars.

L

Linoleic acid – unsaturated Omega-6 fatty acid and is essential to the human diet. It is a component of many vegetables oils, meats, and dairy foods.

Linolenic acid – unsaturated Omega-3 fatty acid and is essential to the human diet. It is a component of some plant oils, fish, and nuts.

M

Macronutrient – a nutrient required by the body in large amount (i.e., protein, carbohydrates, and fats).

Metabolic rate – the amount of energy the body uses in a given timeframe.

Metabolic syndrome – a medical condition that may consist of a combination of diseases (i.e., obesity, high blood sugar, and high blood pressure) that increases risk of heart disease, stroke, and diabetes.

Metabolic waste – the surplus of substances in the body that cannot be used and must be excreted.

Metabolism – the chemical processes by which the body's cells react to substances and energy for sustained life.

Micronutrient – an organic compound needed by the body in small amounts (i.e., vitamins and minerals).

N

Nutrient density – a ratio of nutrient content to the total energy content. Nutrient dense foods provide a substantial amount of nutrients (i.e., vitamins, minerals, and phytonutrients) with relatively few calories.

Nutrient timing – a sports dieting concept that incorporates time as a factor in recovery from training and body composition.

Nutritional age – a level of nutrition knowledge.

O

Obesity – a medical condition in which excess body fat has accumulated to the extent that it places the person at health risk for chronic diseases and shortens the life expectancy. The United States Centers for Disease Control and Prevention classifies a person as obese when he/she has a body mass index of 30 percent or higher.

Overweight – a condition of a person accumulating more body fat than is optimally healthy and can impair movement, flexibility, and overall health that could lead to obesity and chronic diseases. The United States Centers for

Disease Control and Prevention classifies a person as overweight when he/she has a body mass index of 25-30 percent.

P

PH levels – a chemical measure of the acid and alkaline levels within the body. A neutral level is seven, while acidity occurs under seven and alkanility occurs above seven. The body prefers a slightly alkanized state.

Phytonutrients – organic compounds found in plants (i.e., vegetables, fruits, grains, legumes, nuts, and teas) that are thought to promote human health.

Processed foods – foods that have been transformed or modified by methods and techniques to prolong shelf life and make them marketable.

Protein – large and complex compounds that consist of amino acids (i.e., meats, fish, eggs, dairy foods, and some plant-based foods) that are essential for living cells.

R

Refined sugar – raw sugar that has been processed by refining or enhancing its nature. Because refined sugars lack in nutrients and strip the body of nutrient absorption due to its demand on the digestive system, it is considered harmful to health.

Resting metabolic rate – the amount of daily energy expenditure while at rest for the body's vital functions.

S

Satiated – the state of being satisfactorily full from food.

SMART EATS – the 9 principles of healthy eating by the *One Size Does NOT Fit All Diet Plan*.

Specific dynamic action – the thermic effect of food or how the metabolism responds to the digestion of food and the uptake of nutrients in the blood.

Starchy carbohydrates – a group of organic compounds (i.e., grains, tubers, and legumes) that serves as a major energy source in the diet.

Starvation mode – a biological and physiological response that changes and decreases metabolism due to the lack of food.

Supplements – a substance that is taken as food or drink to supplement the diet with nutrients (i.e., vitamins, minerals, fiber, fatty acids, and amino acids) when there are not sufficient amounts provided by the diet through food.

T

Testosterone - a group of steroid hormones that primarily regulate the growth, development, and function of the male reproductive system.

Thermic effect of food – how the metabolism responds to the digestion of food and the uptake of nutrients in the blood.

Thermogenesis – the process of heat production in the body which determines how the metabolism responds to calories burned.

Thyroid – an endocrine gland found in the neck that controls how quickly the body uses energy, makes proteins, and controls the body's sensitivity to other hormones.

Trans fats – unsaturated fatty acids that have been processed through a method called "hydrogenation," changing the chemical structure of the natural fats. Hydrogenation provides a longer shelf life yet creates many health risks such as heart disease, cancer, and other chronic diseases.

U

Unbalanced diet – a diet that does not provide balance with all food groups (i.e., protein, carbohydrate, and fat).

United States Food and Drug Administration (USDA) – the United States government agency that enforces laws on the manufacturing, testing, and use of drugs and medical devices. (It does not regulate dietary supplements.)

W

Weight plateau – a period of stabilization of weight during weight loss or dieting phases.

Index

Endnotes

---

[1] Kohl III, H.W. & Murray, T.D. (2012) Chapter 6: Overweight and Obesity. In Harold W. Kohl, III, and Tinker D. Murray, *Foundations of Physical Activity and Public Health* (pp. 95-116). Location: United States of America.

[2] Berardi, J. & Andrews, R. (2009). Step 3: Evaluating Client Information and Explaining What It Means. International Sports Sciences Association. *Nutrition: The Complete Guide* (307-328). Carpinteria, CA: International Sports Sciences Association.

[3] Centers for Disease Control and Prevention. (2011, May 16). Overweight and Obesity: Causes and Consequences. Retrieved from http://www.cdc.gov/obesity/causes/index.html.

[4] Trust for America's Health. (2011, June). *F as in Fat: How Obesity Threatens America's Future 2010.* Washington, DC: Robert Wood Johnson Foundation. Retrieved from http://healthyamericans.org/reports/obesity2010/Obesity2010Report.pdf.

[5] United States Department of Health and Human Services. (2007, January 11). Overweight and Obesity: Health Consequences. Retrieved from http://www.surgeongeneral.gov/topics/obesity/calltoaction/fact consequences.htm.

[6] The Obese Society. (2008, April 18). Obesity Statistics – U.S. Trends. Retrieved from http://www.obesity.org/statistics/obesity trends.asp.

[7] American Heart Association. (2006, January 11). Heart Disease and Stroke Statistics – 2006 Update. *Circulation, 113*, e85-e151. doi: 10.1161/CIRCULATIONAHA.105.171600. Retrieved from http://circ.ahajournals.org/content/113/6/e85.full.pdf.

[8] Ibid.

[9] National Institute of Diabetes and Digestive and Kidney Diseases. (2007, October). Do You Know the Health Risks of Being Overweight? *WIN – Weight-Control Information Network, NIH Publication No. 07-4098.* Retrieved from http://win.niddk.nih.gov/publications/PDFs/hlthrisks1104.pdf.

[10] United States Department of Health and Human Services. (2001, December). *The Surgeon's Call to Action to Prevent and Decrease Overweight and Obesity* [Data file]. Retrieved from http://www.surgeongeneral.gov/library/calls/obesity/index.html.

[11] Centers for Disease Control and Prevention. (2005, May 25). *Obesity in the News: Helping Clear the Confusion* [Power point presentation].

[12] American Cancer Society. (2007). *Global Cancer Facts and Figures.* Retrieved from http://www.cancer.org/acs/groups/content/@nho/documents/document/globalfactsandfigures2007rev2p.pdf.

[13] United States Department of Health and Human Services. (2001, December). *The Surgeon General's Call to Action to Prevent and Decrease Overweight and Obesity* [Data file]. Retrieved from http://www.surgeongeneral.gov/library/calls/obesity/index.html.

[14] National Institute of Diabetes and Digestive and Kidney Diseases. (2007, October). Do You Know the Health Risks of Being Overweight? *WIN – Weight-Control Information Network, NIH Publication No. 07-4098*. Retrieved from http://win.niddk.nih.gov/publications/PDFs/hlthrisks1104.pdf.

[15] Cowie, C.C., Rust, K.F. & Byrd-Hold, D.D., et al. (2006, June). Prevalence of Diabetes and Impaired Fasting Glucose in Adults in the U.S. Population: National Health and Nutrition Examination Survey 1999-2002. *Diabetes Care, 29(6),* 1263-1268. doi: 10.2337/dc06-0062. Retrieved from http://care.diabetesjournals.org/content/29/6/1263.full.pdf.

[16] Centers for Disease Control and Prevention. (2005, March). *CDC Protecting Health for Life: The State of the CDC Fiscal Year 2004*. Retrieved from http://www.cdc.gov/cdc.pdf.

[17] Wang, Y., Chen, X. & Song, Y., et al. (2008, January). Association between Obesity and Kidney Disease: A Systematic Review and Meta-Analysis. *Kidney Int., 73(1),* 19-33.

[18] United States Department of Health and Human Services. (2001, December). *The Surgeon General's Call to Action to Prevent and Decrease Overweight and Obesity* [Data file]. Retrieved from http://www.surgeongeneral.gov/library/calls/obesity/index.html.

[19] Centers for Disease Control and Prevention. (2010, October 20). *NHIS Arthritis Surveillance*. Retrieved from http://www.cdc.gov/arthritis/data_statistics/national_nhis.htm.

[20] United States Department of Health and Human Services. (2001, December). *The Surgeon General's Call to Action to Prevent and Decrease Overweight and Obesity* [Data file]. Retrieved from http://www.surgeongeneral.gov/library/calls/obesity/index.html.

[21] Beydoun, M.A., Beydoun, H.A. & Wang, Y. (2008, May). Obesity and Central Obesity as Risk Factors for Incident Dementia and Its Subtypes. *Obesity Reviews, 9(3),* 204-218.

[22] Petry, N.M., Barry, D. & Pietrzak, R.H., et al. (2008). Overweight and Obesity Are Associated With Psychiatric Disorders: Results from the National Epidemiological Survey on Alcohol and Related Conditions. *Psychosomatic Medicine, 70,* 288-297. doi: 10.1097/PSY.06013e3181651641. Retrieved from http://www.psychosomaticmedicine.org/content/70/3/288.full.pdf.

[23] United States Department of Health and Human Services. (2001, December). *The Surgeon General's Call to Action to Prevent and Decrease Overweight and Obesity* [Data file]. Retrieved from http://www.surgeongeneral.gov/library/calls/obesity/index.html.

[24] Ogden, C.L., Carroll, M.D. & Curtin, L.R., et al. (2010, January). Prevalence of High Body Mass Index in U.S. Children and Adolescents, 2007-2008. *Journal of American Medical Association, 303(3),* 242-249. doi: 10.1001/jama.2009.2012. Retrieved from http://jama.ama-assn.org/content/303/3/242.full.pdf.

[25] Centers for Disease Control and Prevention. (2008, December). *Prevalence of Overweight, Obesity and Extreme Obesity Among Adults: United States, Trends 1976-80 Through 2005-2006*. National Center for Health Statistics E-Stats. Retrieved from http://www.cdc.gov/nchs/data/hestat/overweight/overweight_adult.pdf.

[26] Flegal, K.M., Carroll, M.D. & Ogden, C.L., et al. (2010, January 20). Prevalence and Trends in Obesity Among U.S. Adults, 1999-2008. *Journal of American Medical Association, 303(3),* 235-241. doi: 10.1001/jama.2009.2014. Retrieved from http://jama.ama-assn.org/content/303/3/235.full.pdf.

[27] Trust for America's Health. (2001, June). *F as in Fat: How Obesity Threatens America's Future 2010.* Washington, DC: Robert Wood Johnson Foundation. Retrieved from http://www.rwjf.org/files/research/20100629fasinfatmainreport.pdf.

[28] The Office of Minority Health. (2012, July 9). *Heart Disease Data/Statistics.* Retrieved from http://minorityhealth.hhs.gov/templates/browse.aspx?lvl=3&lvlid=127.

[29] Flegal, K.M., Carroll, M.D. & Ogden, C.L., et al. (2010, January 20). Prevalence and Trends in Obesity Among U.S. Adults, 1999-2008. *Journal of American Medical Association, 303(3)*, 235-241. doi: 10.1001/jama.2009.2014. Retrieved from http://jama.ama-assn.org/content/303/3/235.full.pdf .

[30] United States Census Bureau. (2010, June 22). *Percentage of People in Poverty by State Using 2- and 3- Year Averages: 2004-2006.* Retrieved from http://www.census.gov/hhes/www/poverty/data/incpovhlth/2006/state.html.

[31] Trust for America's Health. (2011, June). *F as in Fat: How Obesity Threatens America's Future 2010.* Washington, DC: Robert Wood Johnson Foundation. Retrieved from http://www.rwjf.org/files/research/20100629fasinfatmainreport.pdf.

[32] Flegal, K.M., Carroll, M.D. & Ogden, C.L., et al. (2010, January 20). Prevalence and Trends in Obesity Among U.S. Adults, 1999-2008. *Journal of American Medical Association, 303(3)*, 235-241. doi: 10.1001/jama.2009.2014. Retrieved from http://jama.ama-assn.org/content/303/3/235.full.pdf.

[33] Ogden, C.L., Carroll, M.D. & Curtin, L.R., et al. (2010, January). Prevalence of High Body Mass Index in U.S. Children and Adolescents, 2007-2008. *Journal of American Medical Association, 303(3)*, 242-249. doi: 10.1001/jama.2009.2012. Retrieved from http://jama.ama-assn.org/content/303/3/242.full.pdf.

[34] Ogden, C.L., Carroll, M.D. & Flegal, K.M. (2008, May). High Body Mass Index for Age among U.S. Children and Adolescents, 2003-2006. *Journal of American Medical Association, 229(20)*, 2401-2405. doi: 10.1001/jama.299.20.2401. Retrieved from http://jama.ama-assn.org/content/299/20/2401.full.pdf.

[35] Centers for Disease Control and Prevention. (2008, December). *Prevalence of Overweight, Obesity and Extreme Obesity Among Adults: United States, Trends 1976-80 Through 2005-2006.* National Center for Health Statistics E-Stats. Retrieved from http://www.cdc.gov/nchs/data/hestat/overweight/overweight_adult.pdf.

[36] Finkelstein, E.A., Trogdon, J.G. & Cohen, J.W., et al. (2009, July 27). Annual Medical Spending Attributable to Obesity: Payer- and Service-Specific Estimates. *Health Affairs, 28(5)*, w822-w831. doi: 10.1377/hlthaff.28.5.w822. Retrieved from http://obesity.procon.org/sourcefiles/FinkelsteinAnnualMedicalSpending.pdf.

[37] Thorpe, K.E. (2009, November). The Future Costs of Obesity: National and State Estimates of the Impact of Obesity on Direct Health Care Expenses. Retrieved from http://www.nccor.org/downloads/CostofObesityReport-FINAL.pdf.

[38] Centers for Disease Control and Prevention. (2005, March). *CDC Protecting Health for Life: The State of the CDC Fiscal Year 2004.* Retrieved from http://www.cdc.gov/cdc.pdf.

[39] Finkelstein, E.A., Trogdon, J.G. & Cohen, J.W., et al. (2009, July 27). Annual Medical Spending Attributable to Obesity: Payer- and Service-Specific Estimates. *Health Affairs, 28(5)*, w822-w831. doi:

10.1377/hlthaff.28.5.w822. Retrieved from
http://obesity.procon.org/sourcefiles/FinkelsteinAnnualMedicalSpending.pdf.

[40] Cawley, J., Rizzo, J.A. & Hass, K. (2007, December). Occupation-Specific Absenteeism Costs Associated With Obesity and Morbid Obesity. *Journal of Occupational & Environmental Medicine, 49(12)*, 1317-1324. doi: 10.1097/JOM.0b013e31815b56a0.

[41] Gates, D.M., Succop, P. & Brehm, B.J., et al. (2008, January). Obesity and Presenteeism: The Impact of Body Mass Index on Workplace Productivity. *Journal of Occupational & Environmental Medicine, 50(1)*, 39-45. doi: 10.1097/JOM.0b013e31815d8db2. Retrieved from http://www.choixdecarriere.com/pdf/6573/2010/Gates2008.pdf.

[42] Burton, W.M., Chen, C.Y. & Schultz, A.B., et al. (1998, September). The Economic Costs Associated With Body Mass Index In a Workplace. *Journal of Occupational & Environmental Medicine, 40(9)*, 786-792.

[43] United States Department of Agriculture Center for Nutrition Policy and Promotion. (1992, August). *The Food Guide Pyramid, Home and Garden Bulletin Number 252*. Retrieved from http://www.cnpp.usda.gov/Publications/MyPyramid/OriginalFoodGuidePyramids/FGP/FGPPamphlet.pdf.

[44] United States Department of Agriculture Center for Nutrition Policy and Promotion, Food Marketing Institute, and International Food Information Council Foundation. (2006). *Your Personal Path to Health: Steps to a Healthier You!* Retrieved from http://www.cnpp.usda.gov/Publications/MyPyramid/print%20materials/MyPyramidBrochurebyIFIC.pdf.

[45] United States Department of Agriculture and Health and Human Services. (2011, June). *Let's Eat for the Health of It, Home and Garden Bulletin Number 232-CP, HHS Publication Number HHS-ODPHP-2010-01-DGAB*. Retrieved from http://www.choosemyplate.gov/food-groups/downloads/MyPlate/DG2010Brochure.pdf.

[46] Shin, M., Holmes, M.D., Hankinson, S.E. & et al. (2012, April 7). Intake of Dairy Products, Calcium, and Vitamin D and Risk of Breast Cancer. *Journal of the National Cancer Institute, 94(17)*, 1301-1310. doi: 10.1093/jnci/94.17.1301. Retrieved from http://jnci.oxfordjournals.org/content/94/17/1301.full.pdf.

[47] Liu, R.H. (2003, September). Health Benefits of Fruit and Vegetables Are From Additive and Synergistic Combinations of Phytochemicals. *American Journal of Clinical Nutrition, 78(3)*, 517S-520S. Retrieved from http://www.ajcn.org/content/78/3/517S.full.pdf.

[48] Simopoulos, A.P. (2008, June). The Importance of the Omega-6/Omega-3 Fatty Acid Ratio in Cardiovascular Disease and Other Chronic Diseases. *Experimental Biology and Medicine, 233(6)*, 674-688. doi: 10.3181/0711-MR-311. Retrieved from http://ebm.rsmjournals.com/content/233/6/674.full.pdf.

[49] Siri-Tarino, P.W., Sun, Q., Hu, F.B. & et al. (2010, March). Meta-Analysis of Prospective Cohort Studies Evaluating the Association of Saturated Fat with Cardiovascular Disease. *American Journal of Clinical Nutrition, 91(3)*, 535-546. doi: 10.3945/ajcn.2009.277725. Retrieved from http://www.ajcn.org/content/91/3/535.full.pdf.

[50] Mozaffarian, D., Katan, M.B., Ascherio, A. & et al. (2006, April 13). Trans Fatty Acids and Cardiovascular Disease. *The New England Journal of Medicine, 354(15)*, 1601-1613. Retrieved from http://www.nejm.org/doi/full/10.1056/NEJMra054035.

[51] Avena, N.M., Rada, P. & Hoebel, B.G. (2009, March). Sugar and Fat Binging Have Notable Differences in Addictive-Like Behavior. *The Journal of Nutrition, 139(3),* 623-628. doi: 10.3945/jn.108.097584. Retrieved from http://www.ncbi.nlm.nih.gov/pmc/articles/PMC2714381/pdf/nut139623.pdf.

[52] Sievenpiper, J.L., de Souza, R.J. & Mirrahimi, A., et al. (2012, February 21). Effect of Fructose on Body Weight in Controlled Feed Trials: A Systematic Review and Meta-Analysis. *Annals of Internal Medicine, 156(4),* 291-304. Retrieved from http://annals.org/article.aspx?volume=156&page=291.

[53] Liu, H., Huang, D. & McArthur, D.L., et al. (2010, July 20). Fructose Induces Transketolase Flux to Promote Pancreatic Cancer Growth. *Cancer Research, 70,* 6368-6376. doi: 10.1158/0008-542.CAN-09-4615. Retrieved from http://cancerres.aacrjournals.org/content/70/15/6368.full.pdf.

[54] Insawang, T., Selmi, C. & Cha'on, U., et al. (2012, June 8). Monosodium Glutamate (MSG) Intake Is Associated With the Prevalence of Metabolic Syndrome in a Rural Thai Population. *Nutrition & Metabolism, 9(1),* 50. doi: 10.1186/1743-7075-9-50. Retrieved from http://www.nutritionandmetabolism.com/content/pdf/1743-7075-9-50.pdf.

[55] Morrison, J.F., Shehab, S. & Sheen, R., et al. (2008, February). Sensory and Autonomic Nerve Changes in the Monosodium Glutamate-Treated Rat: A Model of Type II Diabetes. *Experimental Physiology, 93(2),* 213-222. doi: 10.1113/expphysiol.2007.039222. Retrieved from http://ep.physoc.org/content/93/2/213.full.pdf.

[56] Samuels, A. (1999). The Toxicity/Safety of Processed Free Glutamic Acid (MSG): A Study in Suppression of Information. *Accountability in Research: Policies and Quality Assurance, 6(4),* 259-310. doi: 10.1080/08989629908573933. Retrieved from http://www.truthinlabeling.org/l-manuscript.htm.

[57] Blaylock, R.L. (2007, December 13). The Truth about Aspartame. CD.

[58] Gold, M. (2002, January 12). Evidence File #4: Reported Aspartame Toxicity Effects. *Report to the United States Food and Drug Administration.* Retrieved from http://www.fda.gov/ohrms/dockets/dailys/03/Jan03/012203/02P-0317_emc-000199.txt.

[59] Colquhoun, J. & Bosch, L.T. (Producers & Directors). (2012). *Hungry for Change* [Motion picture]. United States: Permacology Production Pty Ltd.

[60] WebMD Medical Reference from Healthwise. (2010, July 16). Hypothyroidism: Topic Overview. Retrieved from http://www.webmd.com/a-to-z-guides/hypothyroidism-topic-overview.

[61] Medical News Today. (2009, August 10). What Is Metabolism? How Do Anabolism and Catabolism Affect Body Weight? Retrieved from http://www.medicalnewstoday.com/articles/8871.php.

[62] Mann, T., Tomiyama, J. & Westling, E., et al. (2007, April). Medicare's Search for Effective Obesity Treatments: Diets Are Not the Answer. *American Psychologist, 62(3),* 220-233. doi: 10.1037/0003-066X.62.3.220. Retrieved from http://motivatedandfit.com/wp-content/uploads/2010/03/Diets_dont_work.pdf.

[63] Farshchi, H.R., Taylor, M.A. & Macdonald, I.A. (2005, February). Deleterious Effects of Omitting Breakfast on Insulin Sensitivity and Fasting Lipid Profiles in Healthy Lean Women. *American Journal of Clinical Nutrition, 81(2),* 388-396. Retrieved from http://www.ajcn.org/content/81/2/388.full.pdf.

[64] Farshchi, H.R., Taylor, M.A. & Macdonald, I.A. (2005, January). Beneficial Metabolic Effects of Regular Meal Frequency on Dietary Thermogenesis, Insulin Sensitivity, and Fasting Lipid Profiles on Healthy Obese Women. *American Journal of Clinical Nutrition, 81(1)*, 16-24. Retrieved from http://www.ajcn.org/content/81/1/16.full.pdf.

[65] Pittman, G. (2012, January). *Frequent Meals Prevent Overeating*. Reuters Health. Retrieved from http://www.health24.com/news/DietFood_News_Feed/1-3420,72310.asp.

[66] Hawley, J.A. & Burke, L.M. (1997, April). Effect of Meal Frequency and Timing on Physical Performance. *British Journal of Nutrition, 77(1)*, S91-S103. Retrieved from http://journals.cambridge.org/download.php?file=%2FBJN%2FBJN77_S1%2FS0007114597000123a.pdf&code=24e5f2304c14f681d4063bbf512011e1.

[67] Farshchi, H.R., Taylor, M.A. & Macdonald, I.A. (2005, January). Beneficial Metabolic Effects of Regular Meal Frequency on Dietary Thermogenesis, Insulin Sensitivity, and Fasting Lipid Profiles on Healthy Obese Women. *American Journal of Clinical Nutrition, 81(1)*, 16-24. Retrieved from http://www.ajcn.org/content/81/1/16.full.pdf.

[68] Thalacker-Mercer, A.E., Fleet, J.C., Craig, B.E. & et al. (2007, May). Inadequate Protein Intake Affects Skeletal Muscle Transcript Profiles in Older Humans. *American Journal of Clinical Nutrition, 85(5)*, 1344-1352. Retrieved from http://www.ajcn.org/content/85/5/1344.full.pdf.

[69] Barr, S.B. & Wright, J.C. (2010, July 2). Postprandial Energy Expenditure in Whole-Food and Processed-Food Meals: Implications for Daily Energy Expenditure. *Food & Nutrition Research, 54*, 5114. doi: 10.3402/fnr.v54:0.5144. Retrieved from http://www.ncbi.nlm.nih.gov/pmc/articles/PMC2897733/pdf/FNR-54-5144.pdf.

[70] Slavin, J.L. (2008). Position of the American Dietetic Association: Health Implications of Dietary Fiber. *Journal of the American Dietetic Association, 108*, 1716-1731. doi: 10.1016/j.jada.2008.08.007. Retrieved from http://download.journals.elsevierhealth.com/pdfs/journals/0002-8223/PIIS0002822308015666.pdf?refuid=S0002-8223%2810%2900245-2&refissn=0002-8223&mis=.pdf.

[71] Institute of Medicine of the National Academics (2005). Energy. National Academy of Sciences. *Dietary Reference Intakes for Energy, Carbohydrate, Fiber, Fat, Fatty Acids, Cholesterol, Protein, and Amino Acids* (114). Washington, DC: The National Academies Press.

[72] Berardi, J. & Andrews, R. (2009). The Macronutrients. International Sports Sciences Association. *Nutrition: The Complete Guide* (166-175). Carpinteria, CA: International Sports Sciences Association.

[73] Institute of Medicine of the National Academics (2005). Energy. National Academy of Sciences. *Dietary Reference Intakes for Energy, Carbohydrate, Fiber, Fat, Fatty Acids, Cholesterol, Protein, and Amino Acids* (114). Washington, DC: The National Academies Press.

[74] Blom, W., Lluch, A. & Stafleu, A., et al. (2006, February). Effect of a High-Protein Breakfast on the Postprandial Ghrelin Response. *The American Journal of Clinical Nutrition, 83(2)*, 211-220. Retrieved from http://www.ajcn.org/content/83/2/211.full.pdf.

[75] Yakar, S., Rosen, C.J. & Bemer. W.G., et al. (2002, September 15). Circulating Levels of IGF-1 Directly Regulate Bone Growth and Density. *The Journal of Clinical Investigation, 110(6),* 771-781. doi: 10.1172/JCI15463. Retrieved from http://www.jci.org/articles/view/15463.

[76] Sjogren, K., Leung, K. & Kaplan W., et al. (2007, April 24). Growth Hormone Regulation of Metabolic Expression in Muscle: A Microarray Study in Hypopituitary Men. *American Journal of Physiology Endocrinology and Metabolism, 293(1),* E364-E371. doi: 10.1152/ajpendo.00054.2007. Retrieved from http://ajpendo.physiology.org/content/293/1/E364.full.pdf.

[77] Ibid.

[78] Tipton, K.D., Elliott, T.A. & Cree, M.G., et al. (2004, December). Ingestion of Casein and Whey Proteins Result in Muscle Anabolism after Resistance Exercise. *Medicine & Science in Sports & Exercise, 36(12),* 2073-2081. doi: 10.1249/01.MSS.0000147582.99810.C5. Retrieved from http://www.sportsnutritionworkshop.com/Files/18.SPNT.pdf.

[79] Willett, W.C. (2010, April 6). Fruits, Vegetables, and Cancer Prevention: Turmoil in the Produce Section. *Journal of the National Cancer Institute, 102(8),* 510-511. doi: 10.1093/jnci/djq098. Retrieved from http://jnci.oxfordjournals.org/content/102/8/510.full.pdf.

[80] Ness, A.R. & Powles, J.W. (1997). Fruit and Vegetables, and Cardiovascular Disease: A Review. *International Journal of Epidemiology, 26(1),* 1-13. doi: 10.1093/ije/26.1.1. Retrieved from http://ije.oxfordjournals.org/content/26/1/1.full.pdf.

[81] Duncan, K.H., Bacon, J.A. & Weinsier, R.L. (1983, May). The Effects of High and Low Energy Density Diets on Satiety, Energy Intake, and Eating Time of Obese and Nonobese Subjects. *American Journal of Clinical Nutrition, 37(5),* 763-767. Retrieved from http://www.ajcn.org/content/37/5/763.full.pdf.

[82] Grunwalk, G.K., Seagle, H.M. & Peters, J.C., et al. (2010, April 10). Quantifying and Separating the Effects of Macronutrient Composition and Non-Macronutrients on Energy Density. *British Journal of Nutrition, 86(2),* 265-276. doi: 10.1079/BJN2001404. Retrieved from http://journals.cambridge.org/download.php?file=%2FBJN%2FBJN86_02%2FS0007114501001684a.pdf&code=32e062ccca3786deae713db408d36660.

[83] Bolton, R.P., Heaton, K.W. & Burroughs, L.F. (1981, February). The Role of Dietary Fiber in Satiety, Glucose, and Insulin: Studies with Fruit and Fruit Juice. *American Journal of Clinical Nutrition, 34(2),* 211-217. Retrieved from http://www.ajcn.org/content/34/2/211.full.pdf.

[84] Bell, E.A. & Rolls, B.J. (2001, June). Energy Density of Foods Affect Energy Intake Across Multiple Levels of Fat Content in Lean and Obese Women. *American Journal of Clinical Nutrition, 73(6),* 1010-1018. Retrieved from http://www.ajcn.org/content/73/6/1010.full.pdf.

[85] Berardi, J. & Andrews, R. (2009). The Macronutrients. International Sports Sciences Association. *Nutrition: The Complete Guide* (149-156). Carpinteria, CA: International Sports Sciences Association.

[86] Slowik, G. (2012, March 22). Fiber: Its Importance In Your Diet. Retrieved from http://ehealthmd.com/content/what-fiber.

[87] Berardi, J. & Andrews, R. (2009). The Macronutrients. International Sports Sciences Association. *Nutrition: The Complete Guide* (149-156). Carpinteria, CA: International Sports Sciences Association.

[88] Liu, S., Willett, W.C. & Stampfer, M.J., et al. (2000, June). A Prospective Study of Dietary Glycemic Load, Carbohydrate Intake, and Risk of Coronary Heart Disease. *American Journal of Clinical Nutrition, 71(6),* 1455-1461. Retrieved from http://www.ajcn.org/content/71/6/1455.full.pdf.

[89] Gross, L.G., Li, L. & Ford, E.S., et al. (2004, May). Increased Consumption of Refined Carbohydrates and the Epidemic of Type 2 Diabetes in the United States: An Ecologic Assessment. *American Journal of Clinical Nutrition, 79(5),* 774-779. Retrieved from http://www.ajcn.org/content/79/5/774.full.pdf.

[90] Lajous, M., Boutran-Ruault, M.C. & Fabre, A., et al. (2008, May). Carbohydrates Intake, Glycemic Index, Glycemic Load, and Risk of Post-Menopausal Breast Cancer in a Prospective Study of French Women. *American Journal of Clinical Nutrition, 87(5),* 1384-1391. Retrieved from http://www.ajcn.org/content/87/5/1384.full.pdf.

[91] Liese, A.D., Roach, A.K. & Sparks, K.C., et al. (2003, November). Whole-Grain Intake and Insulin Sensitivity: The Insulin Resistance Atherosclerosis Study. *American Journal of Clinical Nutrition, 78(5),* 965-971. Retrieved from http://www.ajcn.org/content/78/5/965.full.pdf.

[92] Meyer, K.A., Kushi, L.H. & Jacobs, D.R., et al. (2000, April). Carbohydrates, Dietary Fiber, and Incident Type 2 Diabetes in Older Women. *American Journal of Clinical Nutrition, 71(4),* 921-930. Retrieved from http://www.ajcn.org/content/71/4/921.full.pdf.

[93] Hu, F.B. (2010, April 21). Are Refined Carbohydrates Worse Than Saturated Fats? *American Journal of Clinical Nutrition, 91(6),* 1541-1542. Retrieved from http://www.ajcn.org/content/91/6/1541.full.pdf.

[94] Mayo Clinic. (2009, July 1). Mayo Clinic Study Finds Celiac Disease Four More Times More Common than in 1950s: Undiagnosed Celiac Disease Associated with Nearly Quadrupled Mortality. Retrieved from http://www.mayoclinic.org/news2009-rst/5329.html.

[95] Kraft, B.D. & Westman, E.C. (2009, February 26). Schizophrenia, Gluten, and Low-Carbohydrate Ketogenic Diets: A Case Report and Review of the Literature. *Nutrition & Metabolism, 6(10).* doi: 10.1186/1743-7075-6-10. Retrieved from http://www.nutritionandmetabolism.com/content/pdf/1743-7075-6-10.pdf.

[96] Breen, L., Philp, A. & Witard, O.C., et al. (2011, July 11). The Influence of True Carbohydrate-Protein Co-Ingestion Following Endurance Exercise of Myofibrillar and Mitochondrial Protein Synthesis. *The Journal of Physiology, 589,* 4011-4025. doi: 10.113/jphysiol.2011.211888. Retrieved from http://jp.physoc.org/content/589/16/4011.full.pdf.

[97] Ivy, J.L., Lee, M.C. & Brozinick, J.T., et al. (1988). Muscle Glycogen Storage After Different Amounts of Carbohydrate Ingestion. *Journal of Applied Physiology, 65(5),* 2018-2023. Retrieved from http://www.deepdyve.com/lp/the-american-physiological-society/muscle-glycogen-storage-after-different-amounts-of-carbohydrate-I53asrxeem.

[98] Ivy, J.L., Goforth, H.W. & Damon, B.M., et al. (2002, July 12). Early Postexercise Muscle Glycogen Recovery is Enhanced with a Carbohydrate-Protein Supplement. *Journal of Applied Physiology, 93(4),* 1337-1344. doi: 10.1152/japplphysiol.00394.2002. Retrieved from http://jap.physiology.org/content/93/4/1337.full.pdf.

99 Ferguson-Stegall, L., McCleave, E.L. & Ding, Z., et al. (2011, May). Postexercise Carbohydrate-Protein Supplementation Improves Exercise Performance and Intracellular Signaling for Protein Synthesis. *Journal of Strength & Conditioning Research, 25(5),* 1210-1224. doi: 10.1519/JSC.0b013e3318212db21.

100 Berardi, J. & Andrews, R. (2009). The Micronutrients. International Sports Sciences Association. *Nutrition: The Complete Guide* (149-156). Carpinteria, CA: International Sports Sciences Association.

101 United States Food and Drug Administration. (2012, March 13). Trans Fat. Retrieved from http://www.fda.gov/Food/ucm292278.htm?utm_campaign=Google2&utm_source=fdaSearch&utm_medium=website&utm_term=trans%20fats&utm_content=3.

102 Mozaffarian, D., Katan, M.B. & Ascherio, A., et al. (2006, April 13). Trans Fatty Acids and Cardiovascular Disease. *The New England Journal of Medicine, 354,* 1601-1613.

103 Grimm, M.O.W., Rothhaar, T.L. & Grosgen, S., et al. (2011, June 29). Trans Fatty Acids Enhance Amyloidogenic Processing of Alzheimer Amyloid Precursor Protein (APP). *The Journal of Nutritional Biochemistry.* doi: 10.1016/jnutbio.2011.06.015.

104 Hu, J., Vecchia, C.L. & de Groh, M., et al. (2011, November). Dietary Trans Fatty Acids and Cancer Risk. *European Journal of Cancer Prevention, 20(6),* 530-538. doi: 10.1097/CEJ.0b013e328348fbfb.

105 Golomb, B.A., Evans, M.A. & White, H.L., et al. (2012, January 22). Trans Fat Consumption and Aggression. *PLoS ONE, 7(3),* e32175. doi: 10.1371/journal.pone.0032175. Retrieved from http://www.plosone.org/article/info%3Adoi%2F10.1371%2Fjournal.pone.0032175.

106 United States Government Printing Office. (2003, July 11). Food Labeling; Trans Fatty Acids in Nutrition Labeling; Consumer Research to Consider Nutrient Content and Health Claims and Possible Footnote or Disclosure Statements; Final Rule and Proposed Rule. *Federal Register, 68(133),* 41433-41506. Retrieved from http://www.gpo.gov/fdsys/pkg/FR-2003-07-11/pdf/03-17525.pdf.

107 Berardi, J. & Andrews, R. (2009). The Micronutrients. International Sports Sciences Association. *Nutrition: The Complete Guide* (157-165). Carpinteria, CA: International Sports Sciences Association.

108 University of Maryland Medical Center. (2011, May 10). Omega-3 Fatty Acids. Retrieved from http://www.umm.edu/altmed/articles/omega-3-000316.htm/.

109 Gonzalez-Periz, A., Horrillo, R. & Ferre, N., et al. (2009, February 11). Obesity-Induced Insulin Resistance and Hepatic Steatosis are Alleviated by Omega-3 Fatty Acids: A Role for Resolvins and Protectins. *The FASEB Journal, 23(6),* 1946-1957. doi: 10.1096/fj.08-125674. Retrieved from http://www.fasebj.org/content/23/6/1946.full.pdf.

110 Coreet, C., Delarue, J. & Ritz, P., et al. (1997, July 22). Effect of Dietary Fish Oil on Body Fat Mass and Basal Fat Oxidation in Healthy Adults. *International Journal of Obesity, 21,* 632-643. doi: 10.1038/sj.ijo.0800451. Retrieved from http://www.nature.com/ijo/journal/v21/n8/pdf/0800451a.pdf.

111 Berardi, J. & Andrews, R. (2009). Water and Fluid Balance. International Sports Sciences Association. *Nutrition: The Complete Guide* (207-224). Carpinteria, CA: International Sports Sciences Association.

[112] Dennis, E.A., Dengo, A.L. & Comber, D.L., et al. (2010, February). Water Consumption Increases Weight Loss During a Hypocaloric Diet Intervention in Middle-Aged and Older Adults. *Obesity, 18(2)*, 300-307. doi: 10.1038/oby.2009.235. Retrieved from http://www.ipwr.org/documents/WaterWeightLoss.Obesity.2009.pdf.

[113] Han, C. (2011, November). Studies on Tea and Health. *Wei Sheng Yan Jiu, 40(6)*, 802-805.

[114] Serafini, M., Del Rio, D. & Yao, D.N., et al. (2011). Health Benefits of Tea. Benzie, I.F.F. & Wachtel-Galor, S. *Herbal Medicine: Biomolecular and Clinical Aspects* (239-262). Boca Raton, FL: Taylor and Francis Group, LLC.

[115] Auvichayapat, P., Prapochanung, M. & Tunkamnerdthai, O., et al. (2008, February 27). Effectiveness of Green Tea on Weight Reduction in Obese Thais: A Randomized, Controlled Trial. *Physiology & Behavioral 93(3)*, 486-491. doi: 10.1016/j.physbeh2007.10.009.

[116] Behar, J. (2011, December 15). Top 20 Reasons Why 95% of All Diets Fail. Retrieved from http://www.mybesthealthportal.net/nutrition/weight-management/top-20-reasons-why-95-of-all-diets-fail.html.

[117] Berardi, J.M. (2012, June 30). Precision Nutrition Strategies for Success. Retrieved from http://www.precisionnutrition.com/strategies.pdf.

[118] United State Department of Agriculture & United States Department of Health and Human Services. (2010). Balancing Calories to Manage Weights. United State Department of Agriculture & United States Department of Health and Human Services. *Dietary Guidelines for Americans 2010* (8-19). Washington, DC: United States Government Printing Office. Retrieved from http://www.cnpp.usda.gov/Publications/DietaryGuidelines/2010/PolicyDoc/Chapter2.pdf.

[119] Johnston, C.S., Day, C.S. & Swan, P.D. (2002, February). Postprandial Thermogenesis Is Increased 100% on a High-Protein, Low-Fat Diet Versus a High-Carbohydrate, Low-Fat Diet in Healthy Young Women. *Journal of the American College of Nutrition, 21(1)*, 55-61. Retrieved from http://www.jacn.org/content/21/1/55.full.pdf.

[120] Ibid.

[121] Pasiakos, S.M., Vislocky, L.M. & Carbone, J.W., et al. (2010, April). Acute Energy Deprivation Affects Skeletal Muscle Protein Synthesis and Associate Intracellular Signaling Proteins in Physically Active Adults. *The Journal of Nutrition, 140(4)*, 745-751. doi: 10.3945/jn109.118372. Retrieved from http://jn.nutrition.org/content/140/4/745.full.pdf.

[122] Ibid.

[123] Hargreaves, M. (2004). Muscle Glycogen and Metabolic Regulation. *Proceedings of the Nutrition Society, 63(2)*, 217-220. doi: 10.1079/PNS2004344. Retrieved from http://journals.cambridge.org/download.php?file=%2FPNS%2FPNS63_02%2FS0029665104000266a.pdf&code=972d4e40f11319a6b1a15cd526574854.

[124] Chakravarthy, M.V., Pan, Z. & Zhu, Y., et al. (2005, May). "New" Hepatic Fat Activates PRARa to Maintain Glucose, Lipid, and Cholesterol Homeostasis. *Cell Membrane, 1(5)*, 309-322. doi: 10.1016/j.cmet.2005.04.002. Retrieved from http://ac.els-cdn.com/S1550413105001105/1-s2.0-S1550413105001105-

main.pdf?_tid=c9fdad5c6789d894c85256c420b679a0&acdnat=1343078969_01e17680a1f54930f9f939959cf5a517 .

125 Fife, Bruce (Producer). (2009, March 18). Why Hydrogenated Vegetable Oils are Bad for Your Health. *The iHealthTube Newsletter*. Podcast retrieved from http://www.ihealthtube.com/aspx/viewvideo.aspx?v=1875d35d45c4bde1 .

126 Berardi, J. & Andrews, R. (2009). Step 5: Offering Nutritional Supplement Strategies. International Sports Sciences Association. *Nutrition: The Complete Guide* (365-380). Carpinteria, CA: International Sports Sciences Association.

127 Gastelu, D. & Hatfield, F.C. (2010). Chapter 4: Proteins and Amino Acids. International Sports Sciences Association. *Sports Nutrition* (41-65). Carpinteria, CA: International Sports Sciences Association.

128 Berardi, J. & Andrews, R. (2009). Step 5: Offering Nutritional Supplement Strategies. International Sports Sciences Association. *Nutrition: The Complete Guide* (365-380). Carpinteria, CA: International Sports Sciences Association.

129 Gastelu, D. & Hatfield, F.C. (2010). Chapter 8: Minerals. International Sports Sciences Association. *Sports Nutrition* (119-135). Carpinteria, CA: International Sports Sciences Association.

130 Ibid.

131 Ibid.

132 Ibid.

133 Gastelu, D. & Hatfield, F.C. (2010). Chapter 6: Water and Oxygen. International Sports Sciences Association. *Sports Nutrition* (76-97). Carpinteria, CA: International Sports Sciences Association.

20984833R00154

Made in the USA
Lexington, KY
01 March 2013